GROW YOUR OWN DRUGS

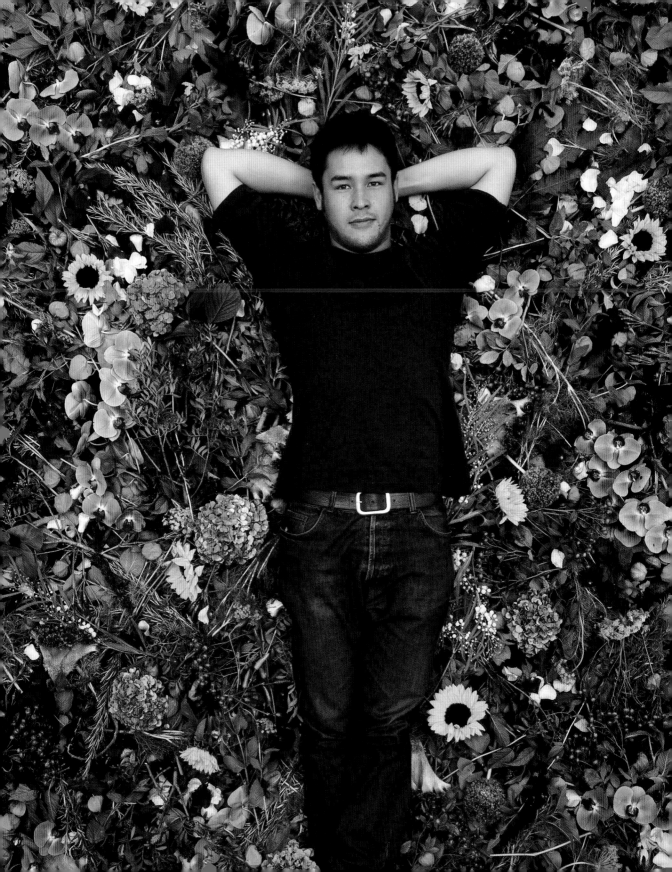

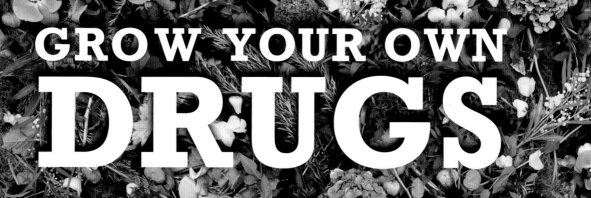

GROW YOUR OWN
DRUGS

Easy recipes for natural remedies and beauty fixes

JAMES WONG

Thorsons

Thorsons
An imprint of HarperCollins*Publishers*
1 London Bridge Street
London SE1 9GF

www.harpercollins.co.uk

First published by Collins 2009
This edition published by Thorsons 2016

12

Text © Silver River Productions Limited 2009
Commissioned photography © Noel Murphy 2009

A catalogue record for this book is available from the British Library.

ISBN 978-0-00-730713-5

Text by Jane Phillimore

Commissioned Photography – Noel Murphy
Design and Art Direction – Smith & Gilmour
Editor – Caroline Curtis
Food Stylist – Annie Rigg
Stylists – Jo Harris, Nel Haynes

Consultant – Liz Williamson, Professor of Pharmacy, University of Reading
Horticultural Adviser – Michael Kerr
Additional recipes by Richard Adams, Hananja Brice-Ytsma and Nathalie Chidley of the
Archway Clinic of Herbal Medicine, and by Liz Williamson
Recipe Testing – Nathalie Chidley

Printed and bound in China

DISCLAIMER
**Please be aware that the advice given in this book is not intended as a replacement for
professional medical treatment and advice. Do not diagnose or medicate yourself or others
without first seeking medical advice. It is advisable to consult a medical practitioner before
using any of these remedies, especially if you have an existing medical condition, are taking
medication, are pregnant or breastfeeding. Some herbs may interact with prescription drugs,
including the Pill and anti-depressants; always do a 24-hour skin test before using. The
publishers and author cannot accept responsibility for any damage incurred as a result
of any of the therapeutic methods contained in this work.**

MIX
Paper from
responsible sources
FSC™ C007454
www.fsc.org

FSC™ is a non-profit international organisation established to promote
the responsible management of the world's forests. Products carrying the
FSC label are independently certified to assure consumers that they come
from forests that are managed to meet the social, economic and
ecological needs of present and future generations,
and other controlled sources.

Find out more about HarperCollins and the environment at
www.harpercollins.co.uk/green

CONTENTS

FOREWORD

To the uninitiated, plants might seem just a bit of frivolous decoration, something to brighten up a windowsill or add a splash of colour to our outdoor spaces. For thousands of kids, being dragged around endless shelves of bedding plants each spring has all the appeal of shopping for soft furnishings. So it's not surprising that my mates think my plant obsession is possibly the least cool of all interests – and looking at it from their perspective, I agree with them.

What none of them realize, however, is that this perception of plants as purely ornamental objects is a strange cultural anomaly that has existed in only one civilization in history – our own. To every other culture, the plants that surround us are a living supermarket, a pharmacy, a builders' merchant and even an off-licence – all rolled into one. In just a couple of generations, we in the West have lost a huge amount of knowledge of the varied and vitally important uses of the botanical world. The irony, however, is that we are just as reliant on plants for all aspects of our daily survival as we have ever been – we just don't know it. They are not only responsible for the air we breath, the food we eat and the stability of the planet's very climate, but are the basis of a large part of our medicine, with up to 50% of the world's top proprietary drugs being originally derived from natural sources.

As an ethnobotanist, I am trained to look beyond the aesthetic and to see plants for what they really are – the chemical factories that make all life on earth possible. When I walk around a garden centre, I see a kind of living pharmacy collected together from all over the world – the leaves of an assassin's poison on one shelf, the flowers of a ritual hallucinogen on another, or a cutting-edge anti-malarial growing as a weed in the pot of a common garden tree that is currently being analysed for use in the treatment of cancer. Looked at this way, plants become warehouses of infinite possibility. Understanding the medicinal uses of the plants around us is not some superhuman (or should that be supergeeky?) ability but is actually the way in which every other culture on earth sees plants – the way, in fact, that we all did until a few short decades ago.

Many of these beliefs aren't just old wives' tales, either, a last bit of mumbo jumbo that has yet to be swept away by reason and science. Traditional plant-based remedies have provided modern Western medicine with some of its most important drugs, and are still studied by pharmaceutical companies, offering tip-offs that may lead to new breakthroughs. Indeed, the natural origins behind major drugs such as aspirin, morphine, penicillin, and even the contraceptive pill reveal that 'natural' medicine is not as separate from 'conventional' medicine as it is popularly conceived to be. In fact, the World Health Organization estimates that up to 80% of the world's population relies on plant-based medicine as the key form of healthcare, and actively promotes its use.

In many ways, I feel fortunate that I first experienced plants not as simply decorative but as an intrinsic part of everyday life in rural Malaysia. I remember sitting, fascinated, on the kitchen floor with my grandmother as she poured mixtures of pungent spices and brightly coloured roots from the garden into a huge stone pestle and mortar, then ground them up into a fragrant mush to make tonics – though also I found, to her horror, that it made great makeshift face paint. Her plants and remedies were always to hand, whether it was small bottles of camphor (*Cinnamomum camphora*) and eucalyptus (*Eucalyptus globulus*) oil whipped out of her handbag to take the itch out of mosquito bites at the Chinese New Year firework display, or the bright red orchid (*Bletilla chinensis*) roots lifted from the back yard and boiled up to make a spicy chicken soup when I had a cold. I was always brought up to see plants as solutions in life rather than just a pretty backdrop to it – and it is a glimpse into this way of seeing plants that I hope this book provides.

INTRODUCTION

In the last few years, there's been a surge of interest in using herbs and plants to treat common ailments. Many people consider plant-based remedies to be natural, cheap and less harmful to the body than pharmaceutical drugs, able to ease both everyday and chronic health problems that orthodox medicine finds so difficult to treat.

At least, that's the theory; the reality is not quite so straightforward. Yes, there's a long history of using plants to treat disease, but until the 20th century these were the only medicines available, and the herbal remedies passed down over the generations cannot necessarily be relied upon. There are up to 50,000 plants used medicinally across the globe, and we're constantly bombarded with 'wonder' claims for the latest, often rather pricy, herbal cure. How can you tell which plants work – and which don't? And which can you grow at home?

This book provides some of the answers. First and foremost, it's a guide to help you get the most out of plants and their various properties. It explains how to grow and harvest suitable plants in your back garden, and then make them into simple, effective remedies to treat a range of common ailments. There are over 60 recipes for teas, tinctures, creams, lotions, balms, gargles, cough syrups and sweets – all easy, cheap and fun to make. And just in case your beauty cupboard is looking bare, there are also lots of natural alternatives to your existing beauty products, from moisturizers and lip salves to bath bombs and face packs.

In the second half of the book, the section Top 100 Plants offers first-class horticultural information as well as scientific insights into the plants, flowers, fruits and roots you'll encounter on your herbal journey. How plants can improve health is currently the subject of much scientific analysis. This book distils the knowledge of herbal practitioners with the most up-to-date scientific findings to bring you practical and reliable information about these plants and the natural remedies made from them. The majority of these plants will happily root in your back garden, but I have also included a few exotic, tender specimens because they are

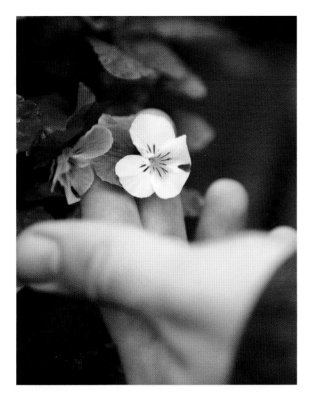
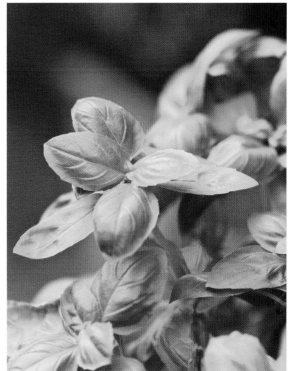
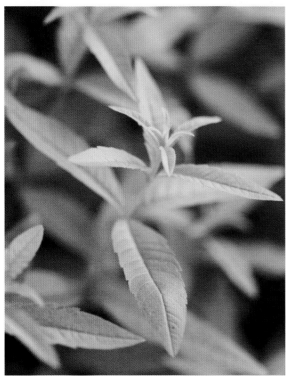
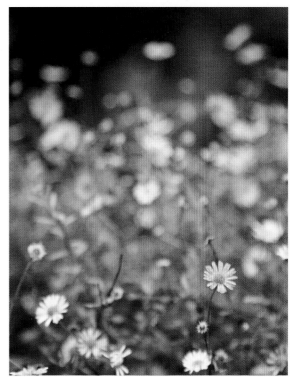

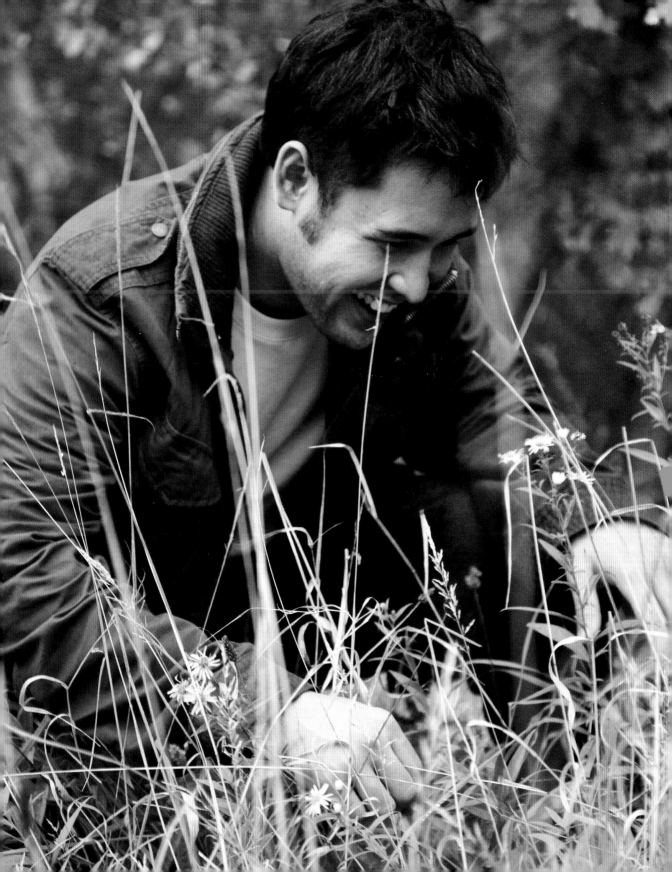

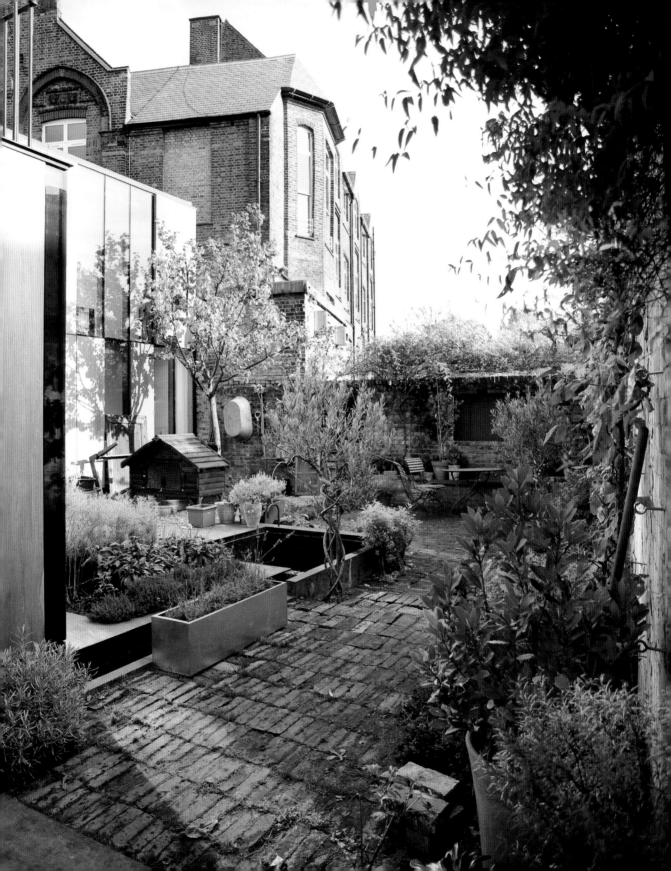

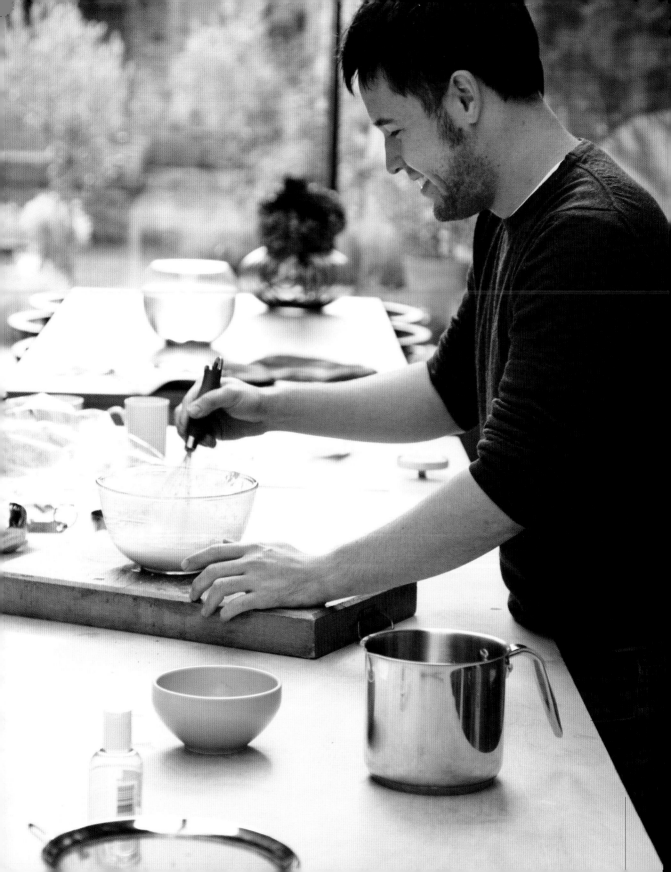

such outstanding performers. You may not be able to grow these yourself, but will find the essential oils or extracts, as well as dried herbs, on sale in health food shops or online.

Safety is a primary concern when using plant material. Although some of these treatments may give over-the-counter medicines a run for their money, it is important that you don't diagnose or medicate yourself or others without first seeking medical advice. This is particularly true if you have an existing medical condition, are taking medication, or are pregnant. Check with your GP before using these remedies. If you think you may be sensitive to any of the ingredients, try a 24-hour skin test first, because some people can react badly to them. Equally important is the need to make sure you have identified the species correctly: certain plants, even those closely related to medicinal species, can be poisonous or deadly.

Using plant-based remedies is a fascinating way to look after your family's health. It's a great pleasure to be in touch with nature, to grow and harvest your own plants, and to make your own remedies. Nowadays, we're lucky enough to have the best of both medical worlds. Modern medicine is hugely effective in the treatment of serious diseases, but plant-based remedies give us gentle ways to manage everyday ailments and keep ourselves in optimum health. You'll never look at your back garden in the same way again.

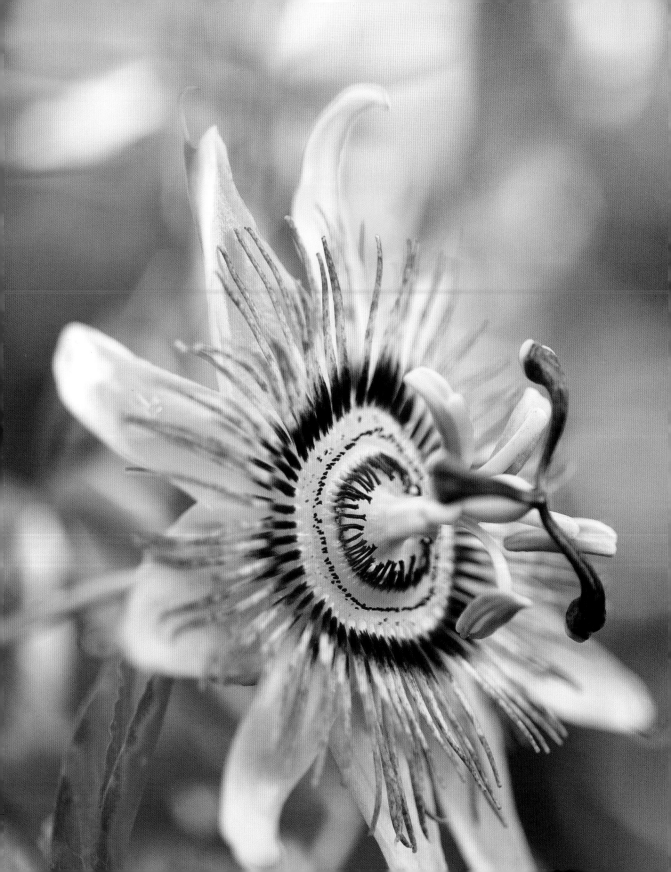

getting started

Reading the labels of the natural remedies and organic cosmetic products found in health food shops, you could be forgiven for thinking that you need to scour the Amazon for rare plants or own a state-of-the-art laboratory to prepare herbal remedies. In reality, however, natural remedies are almost always made from the most common backyard plants, knocked up on the kitchen stove in a matter of minutes.

It is important to remember that traditional plant-based medicine is a system of healthcare that evolved in societies where people did not always have a great deal of money, time or resources. The indigenous women I studied in rural Ecuador as part of the research for my Masters' degree, for example, couldn't go trekking into the mountains for herbs and spend hours grinding, boiling, filtering and drying these each time one of their children has a headache. With up to eight other children to take care of, they needed to find effective solutions in their immediate environment. Solutions that were cheap, easy and quick to prepare – basically made from the contents of their back yard. The parallels with our own time-starved way of life in Western society are obvious.

All you need to get started are the basic tools of any kitchen, as well as access to plant material, whether that's in a tiny window box, your local supermarket or even the weeds growing in your back lawn. Quite literally, if your kitchen facilities and cooking ability can stretch to making beans on toast, you can make herbal remedies. Now go on and get started!

HOME LARDER

Making herbal remedies is just like cooking, and you'll probably find you already have most of the basic ingredients on your kitchen shelves. Staples like olive oil, sea salt, honey, cider or wine vinegar, cornflour and bicarbonate of soda are the basis for many of these recipes. However, there are also a few extra ingredients you'll need, especially if you want to make creams, balms and lotions:

Beeswax and Emulsifying Wax

Lotions and creams are essentially made up of oil and water, but as every schoolchild knows, oil and water don't mix. Something extra – a wax or other emulsifier – is needed to 'glue' and bind the cream together. Emulsifiers work at a molecular level, by attracting and trapping water and oil. They also thicken the mix to create a lotion or cream that can be smoothed into skin.

Beeswax, whether white or yellow, is a natural emulsifier taken from honeycombs, the internal walls of a hive. It is antibacterial, as well as being an excellent skin softener, soother and moisture retainer. You can buy it online as granules, pellets or solid wax. (You can also use beeswax candles or beeswax furniture polish as long as these are labelled 100% pure beeswax.)

Emulsifying waxes are synthetically produced and used in most over-the-counter cosmetic products. There are many different kinds, most of which are suitable for vegans. They usually come as granules, which melt quickly and can be bought online.

Essential Oils

Some recipes use essential plant oils. These add fragrance and many also have medicinal properties – for example, tea tree oil is an antibacterial. However, they are extremely concentrated and should never normally be taken internally. If undiluted oils get on to you skin, wash off immediately.

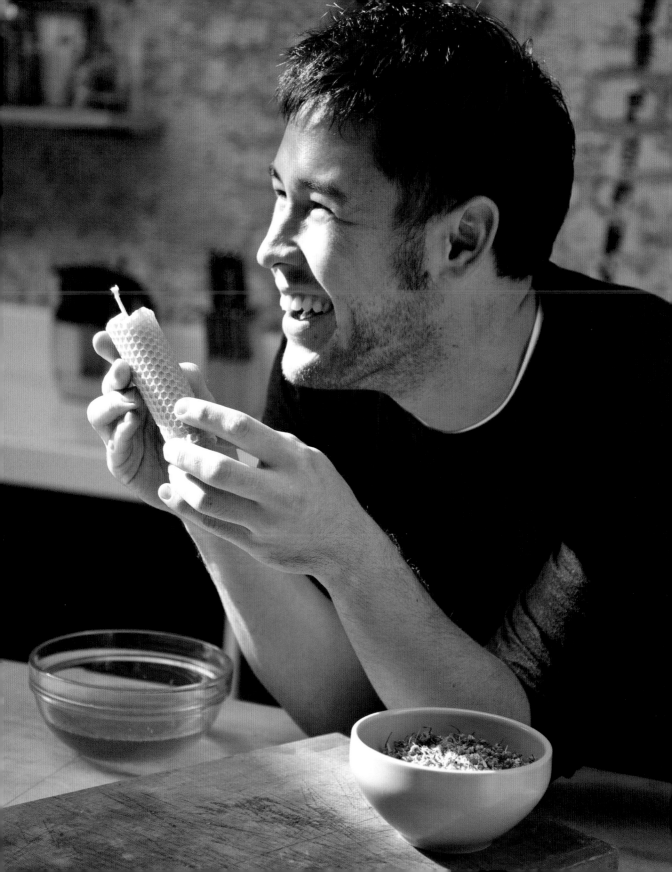

Gelatine

Gelatine is a clear thickening and setting agent used to make gels. Powdered gelatine is easiest to use, dissolved with cold or slightly warm water – boiling water impairs its setting qualities. You can buy animal-based or vegetable gelatine from supermarkets.

Glycerine

Glycerine is a clear, odourless liquid that can be used to make tinctures for children or adults who don't want alcohol-based ones. (Do bear in mind, though, that these tinctures have a shorter shelf life than alcohol-based tinctures). Glycerine is slightly sweet and has soothing properties, so it is often used in over-the-counter products for sore throats and intestinal disorders. It is also used in the preparation of creams, lotions and syrups as a thickener and preserver.

Oils

The base oil for these recipes is usually olive oil, sunflower oil or almond oil (which is good for topical use because it is high in vitamin E). Other oils – such as wheatgerm, avocado, sesame and coconut – have specific properties that are useful in certain remedies. Always choose a fresh, good-quality oil that has been stored in a cool dark place – oils can go rancid quickly.

Vitamin C Powder

Vitamin C is a powerful antioxidant that acts as a natural preservative. It is commonly used in skin creams.

Suppliers

Most of these products are available in supermarkets and health food shops (see Resources, page 219).

OUTDOOR PHARMACY

Where do you find the plants to harvest and make plant-based remedies? You can grow most in your garden at home, and forage others from the countryside, hedgerows and the wild. Many plants used in these recipes grow so freely that they are classed as weeds – chickweed, dandelion, nettles and plantain spring to mind.

Fresh v Dried

Most of the recipes use fresh plant material where possible, so you can grow, pick and use your own directly from the garden, ensuring that all the active ingredients are present in the maximum amounts. However, fresh plant material is unobtainable at certain times of year, so you will have to use dried herbs instead. If these have been dried carefully and thoroughly, they can be used just as effectively as fresh. Drying your own is easy – see How to Dry Plants, page 37. Occasionally dried plants can be a little different to fresh – think of the change in ginger when it is dried – but this is fairly unusual.

When using dried herbs in a recipe, use only about half the amount specified for fresh plant material because it is more concentrated.

Growing at Home

Even if you don't have a garden, you can use pots and window boxes for growing a surprisingly large number of these plants, even small shrubs and trees. For example, a fig tree grows well in a good-sized pot; in fact, restricting its roots in this way makes it produce more and bigger fruit. Plants that do well in pots include:

→ Most small herbs, including caraway, dill, lemon balm, all the mints, parsley and sage.
→ Fruits and vegetables like bilberry, cranberry, goji berries, chilli peppers, garlic, watercress and wheatgrass.
→ Flowers like lavender, marigold (*Calendula officinalis*), nasturtium and rose geranium.
→ Roots like ginger and horseradish.

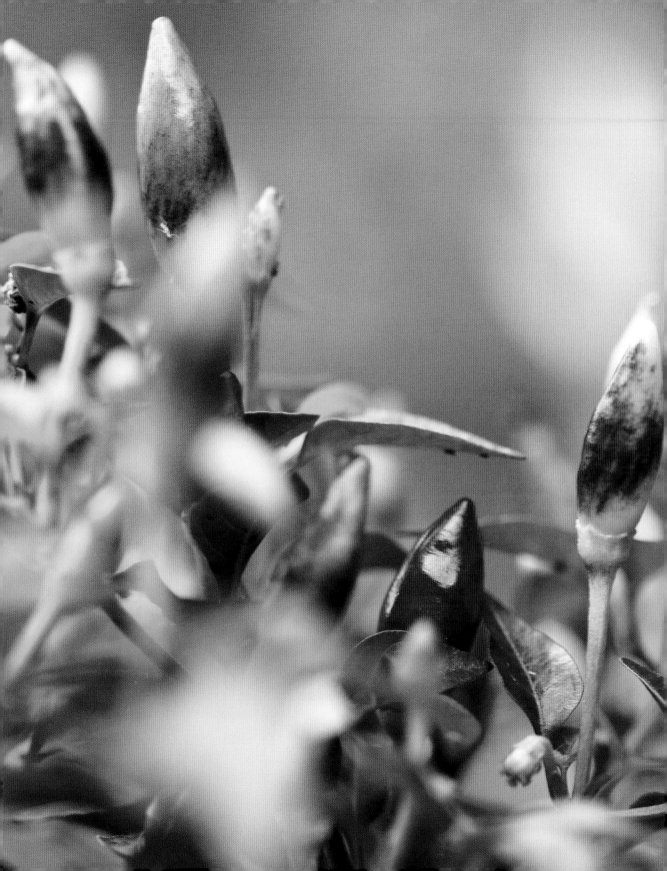

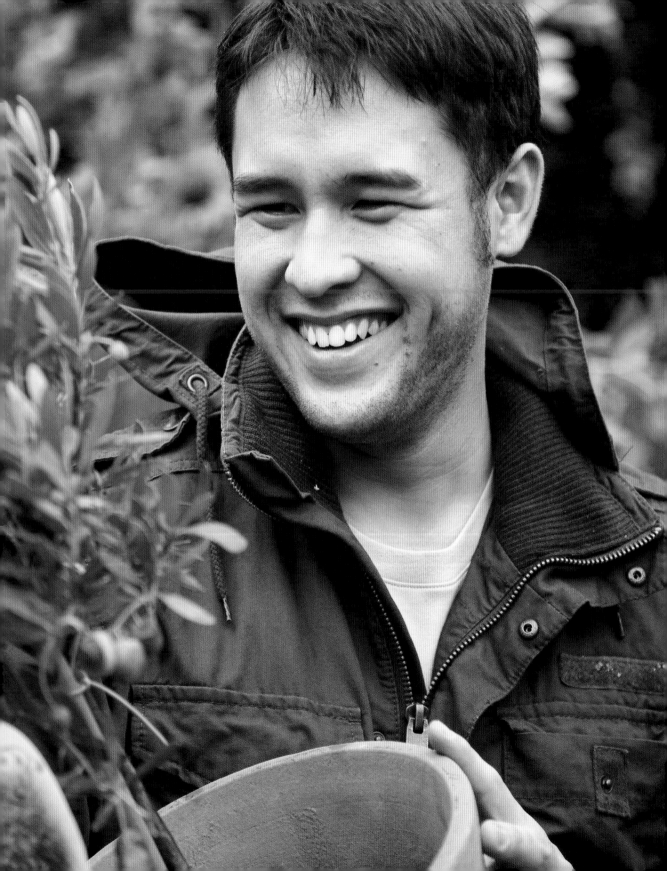

→ Small trees like fig or cultivars of spruce and thuja ('Amber Glow', 'Caespitosa' or 'Tiny Tim'), so long as the pots are large.

The biggest danger with pots is drought: the soil dries out quickly, especially in highly porous terracotta pots, leaving the roots searching round to find water in a very confined space. Water and feed the soil in pots regularly during the growing season from spring to summer, but keep the potting mix from just drying out in winter (overwatering is as big a killer as underwatering in indoor plants). Whenever you can, put pots outside on balconies, porches or window ledges to catch the sun, and choose frost-resistant containers that won't crack and expose roots to freezing temperatures.

TOP 10 SUPERSTAR PATCH

Even in the smallest garden, you can create a complete medicinal herb patch. With space at a premium, you need to make sure that each plant is really earning its keep.

These are the 10 plants that are as versatile as they are effective:

Chamomile (*Matricaria recutita*) – soothes indigestion and colic, eases tension, and is good for skin irritations.

Echinacea – boosts the immune system, and lessens the severity of colds and flu.

Lavender – calms and relaxes, eases pain, and is antiseptic for cuts and bruises.

Lemon Balm – soothes nervous tension and anxiety, promotes sleep, and is good for cold sores.

Marigold (*Calendula officinalis*) – good for sunburn, and for acne and spots, soothes ulcers and digestive problems.

Peppermint – good for digestion, wind and headaches.

Rosemary – helps memory and concentration, improves mood, sweetens breath.

Sage – for coughs, colds and congestion, hot flushes.

St John's wort – anti-depressant and promotes skin healing.

Viola (*Viola tricolor*) – anti-inflammatory, good for eczema and skin eruptions, and loosens phlegm.

If you have a greenhouse, you can boost the contents of your herbal cabinet by growing useful but tender plants such as ginger and cucumber. If you have a windowsill only, an aloe vera plant is a great option.

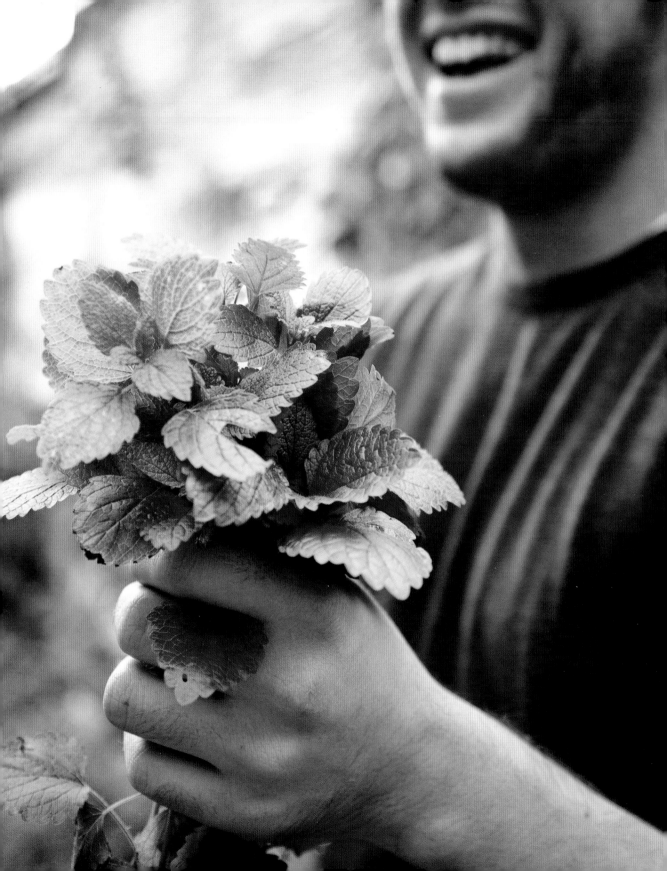

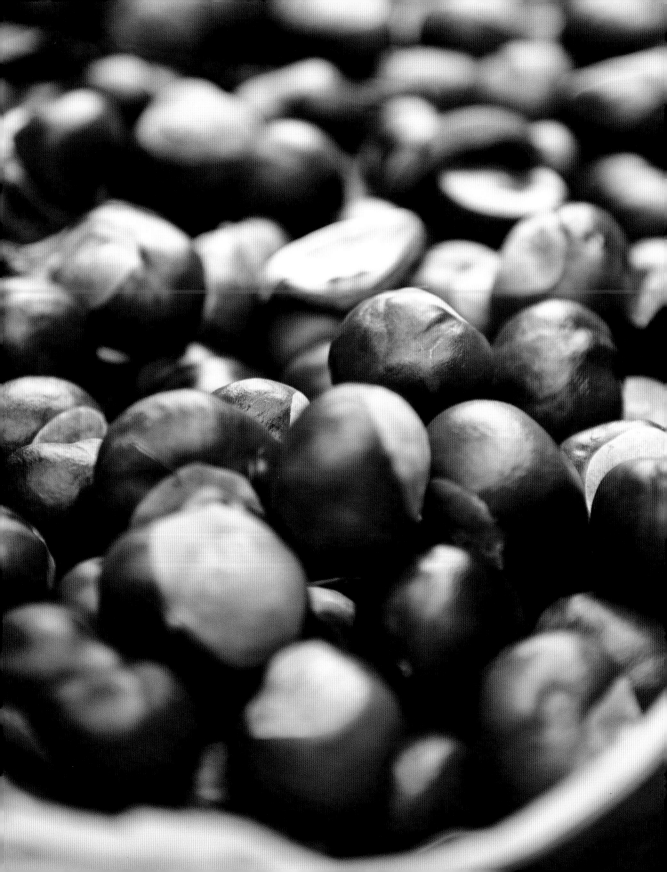

Buying Plants

Most plants can be grown from seed or bought in your local garden centre. Less common plants and trees can be sourced from specialist nurseries or online. Check the Royal Horticultural Sociaty (RHS) plantfinder database (www.rhs.org.uk) for information about nurseries that grow the particular plant you want.

In the Wild

Many of the plants in this book grow plentifully in the countryside or even on wasteland in towns and cities. For example, you can pick up conkers from under horse chestnut trees in your local park in September and October or find elderflowers on wasteland in late May and June.

Best Time for Harvesting

Leaves – gather leaves throughout the growing season (usually spring to autumn). If you want to harvest large amounts of a certain plant, cut back in early summer to half its height, leaving enough regrowth time for a second cutting later in the year.

Flowers – pick as soon as possible after they open.

Roots – harvest in autumn, when roots have most stored food and essential compounds.

Fruits and Seeds – pick when they ripen to a mature colour, before they shrivel or decay.

Plants grow in a variety of habitats in Britain and can sometimes be found in surprising places. It's worth keeping your eyes open for foraging opportunities wherever you are. On a trip to the coast in September or October, you might just spot goji berries and fennel coming into seed. On moorland, especially in Scotland and the north of England, look out for bilberries and juniper berries, while wild thyme loves the chalky downlands of southern England. Hedgerows are good sources of rosehips, haws and sloes, and on rough wasteland you'll often find feverfew, elderflowers and weeds like nettles and dandelion. In woodland, look out for lime flowers and wild garlic.

Foraging Rules

You can gather fruit, flowers and foliage on wild land, so long as it is for your own use and not for resale. Still, there are a few guidelines that should always be followed when harvesting plants:

→ Don't pick something unless you're absolutely sure what it is. It is easy to mix up two plants that look alike or which have similar names; for example, harmless, edible, sweet cicely and toxic hemlock look very similar. Take a well-illustrated field guide with you to identify plants. The Botanical Society of the British Isles (BSBI) has produced various guides, or check against the plant identifications and distribution maps available on its website (www.bsbi.org.uk).

→ Don't pick from beside busy roads or on agricultural land, because the plants are likely to be polluted or sprayed with pesticides and chemical fertilizers. Remember, hedgerows at the edges of cultivated fields may also be in the spray zone.

→ Don't pick plants that look diseased or stunted: you want the healthiest specimens you can find.

→ Harvest only as much as you will use, and don't take more than half the leaves, fruit or stems of any plant. Always leave enough for wildlife to eat and to ensure future plant generations. If there's not enough of a plant to leave some of it behind, then don't pick it.

→ Check with the local landowner before you dig up roots: you have a legal obligation to get permission from them first.

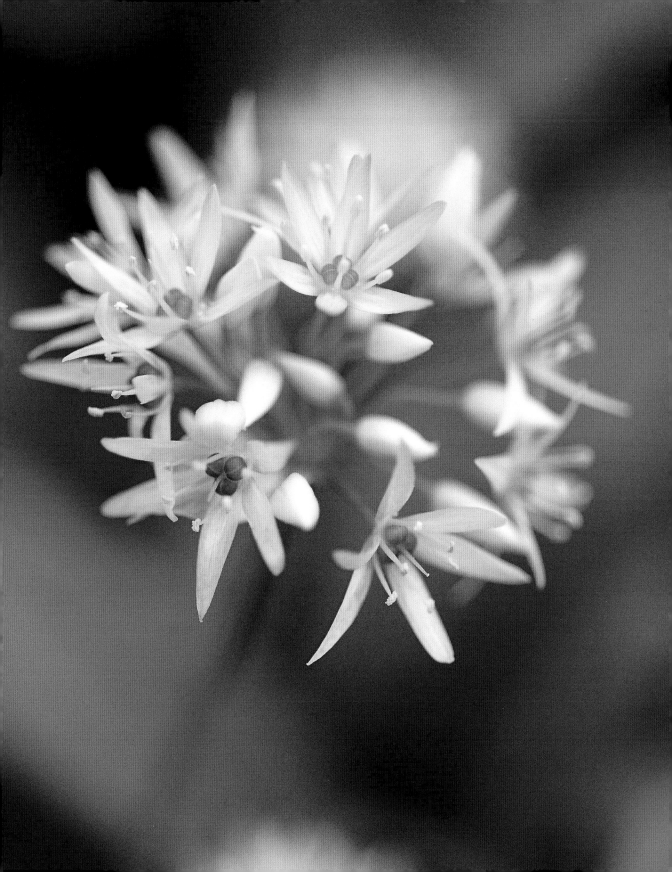

→ Don't dig up roots unless it is a prolific plant, such as dandelion. Don't harvest too many roots in any one area.
→ Never pick a rare or endangered species. You can download a rare plant register from the website of the BSBI (www.bsbi.org.uk).

Foraging Kit

All you need is a bag and a pair of scissors, but foraging fanatics may want to add the following items to their kit:
→ secateurs
→ scissors (for delicate stalks)
→ hand shovel (for roots)
→ knife
→ carrier bags or trugs, to carry stems, flowers and leaves
→ paper bags, to keep seeds dry and cool
→ sealed plastic containers, to prevent fruit from squashing
→ gardening gloves

Remember to keep your arms and legs covered to avoid nettle stings, insect bites and thorns. Good luck!

USEFUL KIT

You don't need any special equipment for making these remedies, though a few kitchen utensils will come in handy:
→ a teapot with a lid, to make tisanes and infusions
→ weighing scales
→ a measuring jug
→ glass mixing bowls of various sizes
→ saucepans
→ a fine-meshed sieve; colander
→ blender
→ whisk
→ wooden and large metal spoons

You may also find the following handy:

Mortar and Pestle – leaves, roots and seeds should be as fresh as possible, so it's always best to grind your own. You can use a mortar and pestle, or even a hand-propelled coffee grinder or pepper mill. But keep the grinder just for this use, or both the ground herbs and the coffee/pepper will taste awful.

Pan and Glass Bowl – plants, oils and waxes need to be heated slowly and evenly and the best way to do this is in a double boiler or bain-marie. This is essentially a pan in which water is heated, with a bowl placed on top which holds the ingredients. Beeswax can leave nasty residues, so if you're making regular batches of creams you may want to invest in a dedicated pan and bowl set.

Muslin or Cheesecloth – invaluable for straining herbs. Use a double thickness to line a sieve or colander and then strain infusions and oils through it. Squeeze out excess juice by twisting the muslin in your hands.

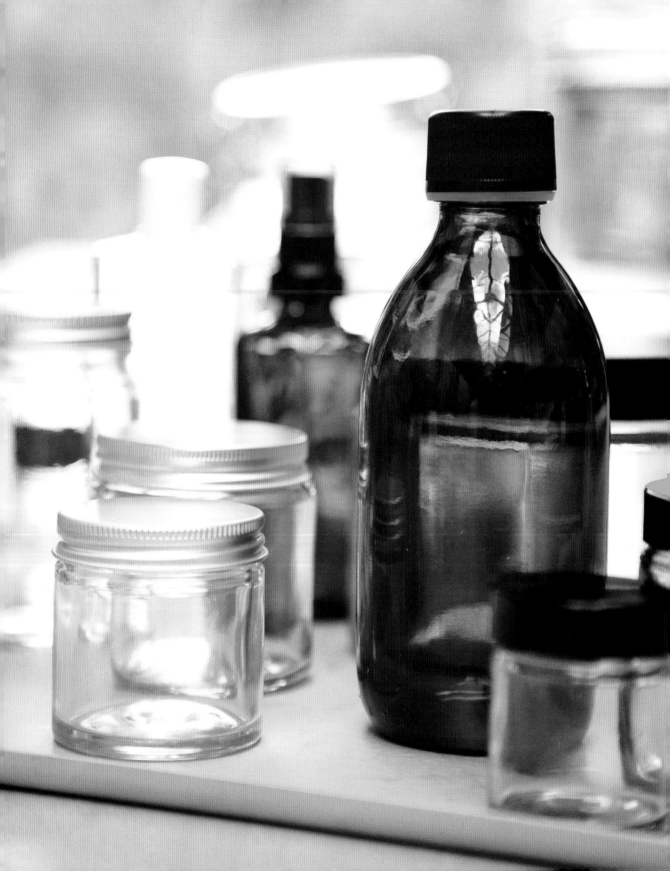

Glass Jars – of all shapes and sizes, new or recycled. Kilner or other canning jars with tight-fitting lids are good for macerating oils; Winchester and syrup bottles for storing syrups and linctuses; and small, wide-mouthed balm jars for salves and ointments. You can get screw, stopper and spray tops, or pipette and dropper tops for tiny dosages. Glass usually comes clear or coloured (amber, blue, brown, black). Clear glass is good for storing herbs (you can easily check for fading and colour changes, signs of deterioration). Dark glass is better for storing oils and tinctures over long periods of time, because it offers protection from the light. Before you bottle a preparation, always sterilize jars. Wash jars and lids in very hot water. Rinse well. Place on a baking tray lined with greaseproof paper. Turn your oven to a low setting (70°C) and place the jars inside. Leave for at least 20 minutes. This will dry and warm them, ready for filling. Alternatively, you can put them through the hottest dishwasher cycle.

Filters and Funnels – getting hot liquid into bottles is easier using these. Metal or plastic filters or funnels work well, and come in various sizes (from cookery shops).

Stick-on Labels – to record the name, date made, dosage, and storage details. It's important not to use treatments after the recommended storage time.

Notebook – to record your experiences, where and when you picked the plants, your favourite recipes, how they helped, suppliers' details, etc.

USING PLANTS

You can take plant-based remedies internally as teas, oils, vinegars and syrups, or use them externally as creams, balms, bath/massage oils, and poultices.

Tea or Infusion – just like making a cup of tea
The simplest way to extract the essential constituents of fresh leaves and flowers is by making an infusion. Place the washed, chopped plants in a glass bowl, pour freshly boiled water over (about 30 g fresh plant to 500 ml water; or 15 g dried plant material). Leave to stand, covered, for 8–10 minutes, or until the water takes on colour. Strain through a sieve lined with muslin. Drink the same day, pour into a bath, or use in lotions and creams.

Decoction – like making tea but left to simmer
Roots, barks and woody parts of the plant need to be left to simmer to extract the essential ingredients, a process called decoction. Wash and chop the root, place in a pan and add water (about 30 g fresh root to 500 ml water). Cover the pan and bring to the boil, then simmer for at least 10 minutes. Strain through a sieve lined with muslin. Drink the same day, pour into a bath, or use in lotions and creams.

Tinctures – chopped plants steeped in alcohol
A tincture uses alcohol to extract the essential compounds from plants. This is highly effective, especially for fibrous plants, roots and resins. Vodka is the alcohol of first choice, being colourless and almost flavourless, but rum, brandy or whisky can also be used. Make sure the alcohol is 80% proof (that is, 40% alcohol), or the tincture may go mouldy in the bottle.

To make a tincture, fill a jar with plant material and cover with alcohol. Run a knife inside the sides to dispel any air bubbles. Seal and leave in a dark cool place for 8 days to 1 month, shaking occasionally. When ready, strain through a muslin-lined sieve and decant into small bottles. Alcohol is a preservative, so tinctures have a longer shelf life than other preparations, keeping for up to 5 years.

Infused Oils – just like making tea but using oil instead of water

Infused or macerated oils – in which plants are left in a base oil for up to 2 weeks to extract their essential compounds – are used to make creams, lotions and massage oils for external or sometimes internal use. To infuse oil, fill a jar with plant material and cover with oil. Run a knife around the inside to dispel air bubbles. Seal and leave in a warm place for 2 weeks, or until the oil has taken on colour, then strain and bottle. For a quicker maceration, place the herbs and oil in a pan and cook over a low heat for about 20 minutes. Strain and bottle. Infused oils will last from 6 months to 1 year.

Salves and Balms

To make a lip salve, ointment or balm, add beeswax to an infused oil and heat gently to melt. The waxy mixture solidifies as it cools. Lip salves and balms are thicker than ointments, which are generally applied over a larger area of the body. Check the mix is the consistency you want by spooning a few drops into a glass of iced water. A thick salve will form into a little ball, a thinner ointment will disperse over the surface. You can thicken by adding more beeswax (½ tsp at a time) or thin by adding more oil (1 tsp at a time), testing again until you get the required consistency. When ready, pour while still warm into wide-mouthed jars for easy use. Salves will last 1–2 years.

Creams and Lotions

These are emulsions, made by mixing a water-based and an oil-based preparation together over heat and 'glueing' them together with an emulsifier like beeswax or emulsifying wax. These are lovely to use on skin, but have a shorter shelf life than salves: they will last in the refrigerator for up to 2 months.

Gels

Used in making skin preparations such as spot gels or face masks. Gels are made by dissolving gelatine with an infusion or juice. Normally used at once, though will keep longer if alcohol or essential oils are added.

Herb-infused Honeys

Honey is an antibacterial agent and can be applied topically to wounds. Herb-infused honeys are very simple to make: simply heat the herbs with the honey for about 1 hour, then bottle. They are often used as throat soothers and to help with congestion in the upper respiratory tract. Naturally sweet, these honeys are a good way to encourage children to take herbs: spread on toast or give a spoonful every day. They will last for up to 6 months.

Syrups and Lozenges

Cough syrups are like runny jams, made by boiling the plant in water with sugar or honey, sometimes with gelatine added as a thickener. They keep well in sterilized jars – from 6 months to 1 year if sealed and unopened; and, once opened, for 3 months in the refrigerator. Adding more sugar or continuing the boiling process, you can produce a solidified mass that can be broken up into small cough sweets, for use throughout the day.

Vinegars

Vinegar also extracts the essential constituents from plants, when heated with the herbs for a few hours. Herbal vinegars can be used in cooking, salad dressings, or taken by spoon every day. They can also be used externally as a hair rinse and tonic, or added to a bath. Cider or wine vinegar are usually used as the base. They will keep for about 6 months or possibly longer.

Poultices and Compresses

The body can absorb essential compounds through the skin, and applying plant material directly as a poultice can relieve backache, muscle pains, strains and headaches, and help to clear skin outbreaks. A simple poultice is made of crushed plants, sometimes mixed in a flour paste. Apply to the skin and cover with gauze and a bandage. Change every few hours.

A compress applies plant infusions or decoctions directly to skin. To make, soak a linen or cotton cloth in the hot or cold plant infusion or decoction. Wring out, then apply. Hot compresses need to be changed regularly.

How to Dry Plants

Drying plants allows you to use them out of season. Dried plants must not contain too much residual water, to avoid spoilage by moulds; they should be dried quickly but without too much heat; and should be kept out of direct sunlight, to avoid destroying the active compounds. There are two methods:

Air Drying – gather loose, leafy bunches of plants, then tie with string or an elastic band. Hang upside down (so the oils go into the leaves), in a well-ventilated, dry environment out of direct sunlight. Leave for at least 2 weeks, or until crispy. When ready, strip the leaves/flowers off, then crumble and store in an airtight coloured glass jar or container. They will keep for up to 1 year.

Oven-drying – cover a baking sheet with greaseproof paper and then put the plants on it, spacing them well apart. Place in the oven on the lowest setting, leaving the door slightly open, until dry – this may take anything up to 5 hours. Crumble and store as above.

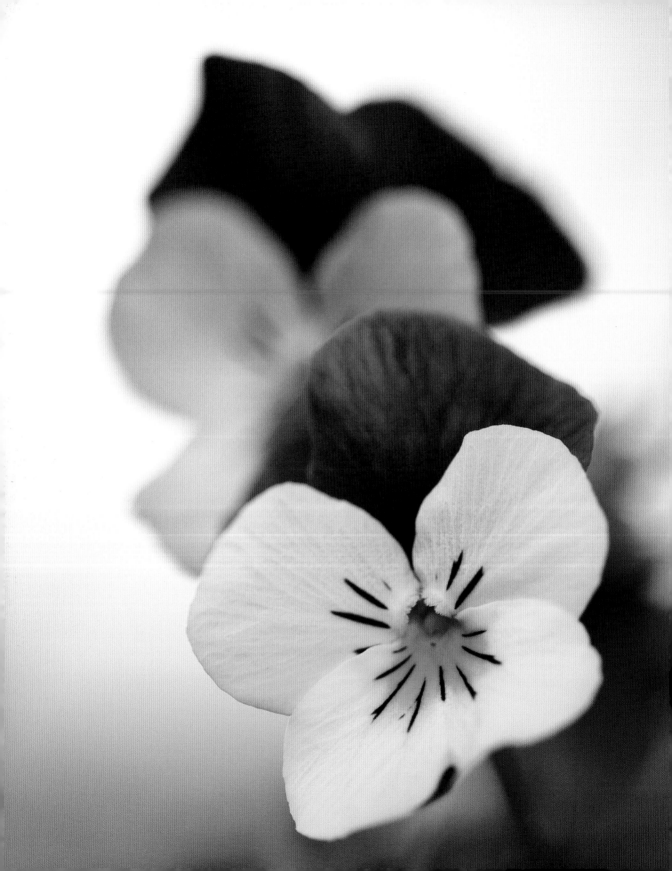

remedies

This is the really fun bit. For me, cooking up these concoctions is like reverting back to childhood, stirring sticky mixtures, pouring out gloopy gels and playing around with amazing smells, colours and flavours. The fact that these remedies might just be effective in clearing up a breakout of acne, calming you down in times of anxiety or even alleviating chronic nausea is almost just an added bonus.

To make things easy for you, we've broken down these recipes according to the type of complaints they treat, and have often given a couple of recipes for each condition so you can experiment to find out what works best for you.

Aside from being fun to make, most are straightforward. Indeed, this section is just like a cookbook. Read through the recipe to check for the ingredients you need and to find out if, for example, it takes a while to macerate (soak) – and then you're all set. It's a great excuse to get the kids involved too: what better way to learn about plants and science than making and explosively fizzy bath bomb?

DIGESTIVE DISORDERS

Bad breath is the scourge of stomach ailments, but thyme is a great healer (excuse the pun). As an essential oil it contains thymol, a powerful antiseptic used in dentistry. Combined with mint and aniseed, two other big odour-busters, it makes an excellent breath freshener.

BAD BREATH
Thyme Sweet Breath Spray and Mouthwash

10 tbsp (approx. 25 g) fresh thyme leaves
10 tbsp (approx. 30 g) fresh mint leaves
5 fresh eucalyptus leaves
3 tsp aniseed
3 tsp cloves
200 ml vodka
rind of 1 lemon
1 tbsp sorbitol or other artificial sweetener to taste, if desired
4 tbsp glycerine

1 Strip the thyme, mint and eucalpytus leaves from their stems and chop. Place in a blender and whiz. Add the aniseed and cloves to the blender and whiz again.

2 Place in a dark bottle with the vodka, lemon and sorbitol (if using) and leave for 10 days to 1 month to macerate.

3 Strain through muslin. Add the glycerine, then stir and pour into a 50 ml spray bottle (with a yield of up to 1 ml per spray).

USE Spray 1 ml into the mouth when needed. NB This contains alcohol, so be careful not to overuse, especially if driving. Do not use if pregnant.
STORAGE Keeps for up to 1 year.

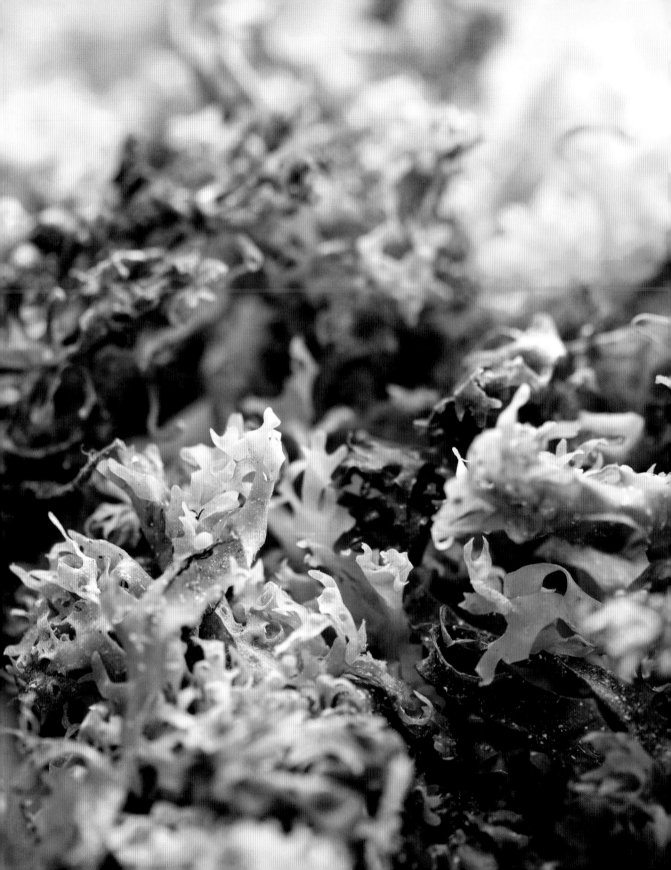

Bloating and belching are unpleasant but very common side effects of heartburn and indigestion. At the first sign of trouble, take a spoonful of this soothing mix. The seaweed coats and protects the stomach lining but also floats on top of the stomach contents, acting as a 'raft' to calm things down and stop reflux. It also works as an antacid, thanks to the bicarbonate of soda.

HEARTBURN AND INDIGESTION

Seaweed Stomach Soother

2 cups Irish moss – *Chondrus crispus* seaweed
(see Resources, page 219)
4 tbsp fennel seeds
4 tbsp mint leaves
500 ml water
125 ml glycerine
4 tbsp bicarbonate of soda

1 Simmer the Irish moss, fennel seeds and mint leaves in the water for 20–30 minutes, or until the liquid has reduced to 250 ml.

2 Blend in a liquidizer with the glycerine until smooth, then strain through a sieve covered with muslin. Leave to cool.

3 Whisk in the bicarbonate of soda, then pour the mixture through a funnel into a sterilized bottle.

USE Take 2 tsp whenever you feel symptoms coming on. See your doctor if symptoms persist for more than a few days.
STORAGE Keeps for 1 month in the refrigerator.

A tasty liqueur that helps with all manner of digestive complaints, including colic, period pains and chills.

DIGESTION
Angelica Tummy Soother

100 g fresh angelica root, chopped
25 g fresh peppermint leaves
125 g fresh juniper berries
750 ml vodka
sugar to taste

1 Put the angelica, peppermint, juniper berries and vodka in a wide-necked bottle or jar with an airtight lid or stopper. Allow to stand in sunlight or in a warm place for 10 days.

2 Strain through muslin and add sugar to taste, then filter into a sterilized bottle or jar.

USE Take a small wineglassful 1–2 times a day when needed.
NB This contains alcohol so be careful not to overuse, especially if driving. Do not use if pregnant.
STORAGE Keeps well for up to 6 months.

Menthol found in mint leaves is used in commercial preparations to treat Irritable Bowel Syndrome. An alternate way to take it is by simply making a cup of mint tea. It can also alleviate wind, colic, indigestion and heartburn.

IRRITABLE BOWEL SYNDROME
Peppermint Tea

1 tbsp fresh peppermint leaves
1 drinking cup hot water

Steep the leaves in hot water for 5 minutes.
Drink whenever needed.

Senna (*Senna alexandrina*) has been used for centuries as a safe and highly effective laxative. I've used the pods, which have a gentler effect than the leaves. Adding figs provides soluble fibre to help digestion and soothe the gut, thus preventing griping. This syrup will quickly relieve the discomfort of constipation. It is best taken before bed, as it takes 8–12 hours to have its effect.

CONSTIPATION
Syrup of Figs

18 g dried senna pods
100 ml boiling water
8 fresh figs, quartered
100 g sugar
juice of 1 lemon

1 Place the senna pods in a glass bowl and pour over the boiling water. Leave to steep for about 30 minutes, then strain through a sieve or piece of muslin into a blender.

2 Add the figs and sugar to the senna infusion and whiz until smooth.

3 Pour into a saucepan, and heat slowly to reduce, stirring occasionally. You want to end up with a thick, glossy sugar-like syrup – this will probably take about 25 minutes. Add the lemon juice and stir in well.

4 Take off the heat and pour the syrup into a sterilized 150 ml bottle.

USE Shake well before use. Take 2 tsp before bed when needed. Don't use for more than a few days at a time, or if you have severe abdominal pain.
STORAGE Keeps in the refrigerator for 3–4 weeks.

VARIATION
Senna and Ginger Tea

Senna can have a cloying, slightly unpleasant taste and mixing it with ginger makes it more palatable, as well as relaxing muscles in the gut to prevent cramping. Take 1 tsp dried senna pods, add 2 cm ginger root, peeled and chopped, and pour over 250 ml freshly boiled water. Leave for 10 minutes to infuse. Strain. You can add a squeeze of lemon juice if you like. Drink while still warm before bed.

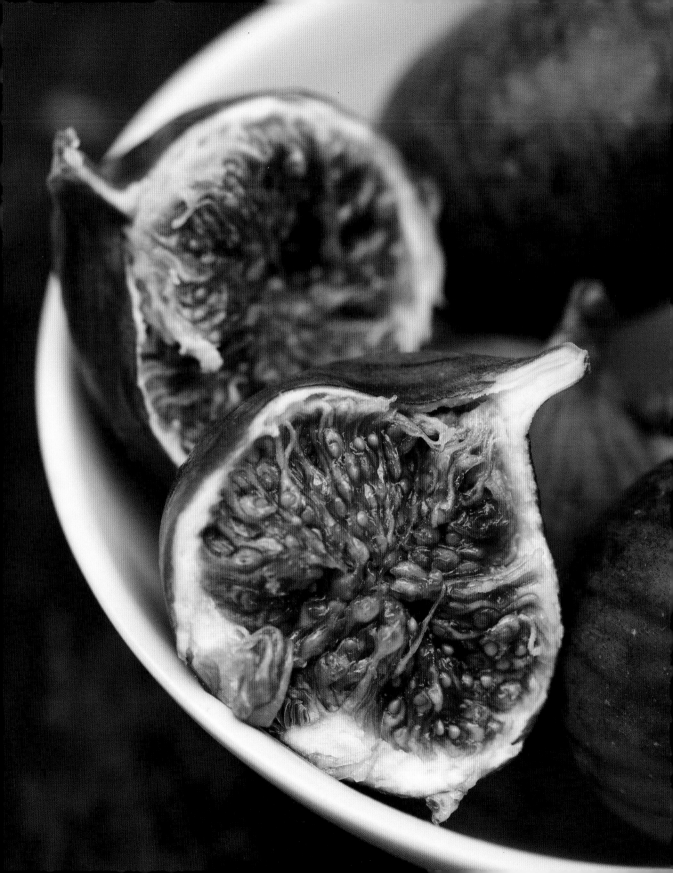

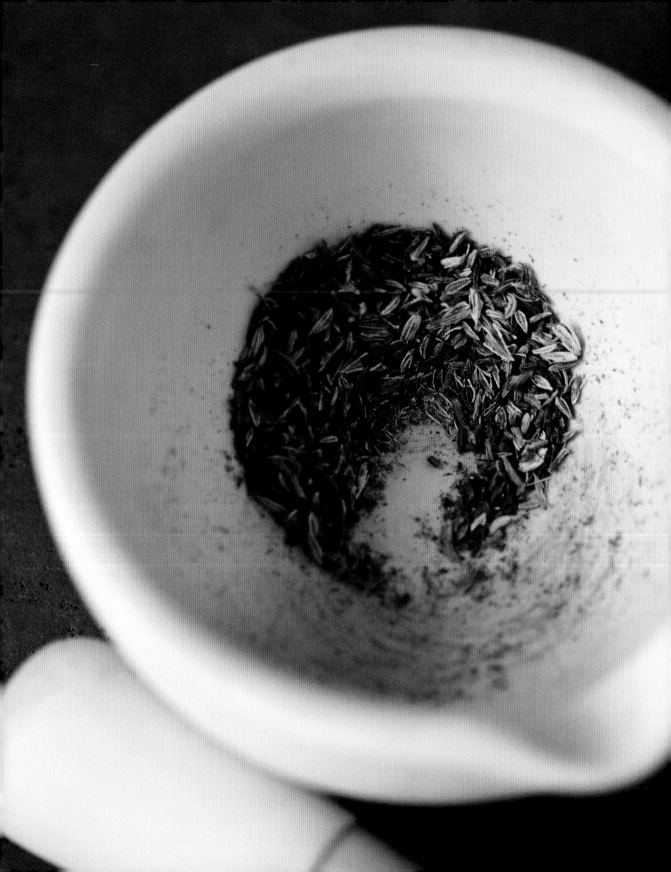

A fresh, tangy brew with four ingredients that all work to release trapped intestinal wind – which may explain its name. The herbs have an anti-spasmodic effect that relaxes the gut, so gas escapes and bloating is relieved.

FLATULENCE

'Four Winds' Tea

1 tsp caraway seeds
1 tsp fennel seeds
1 tsp chopped peppermint leaves
1 tsp chamomile flowers
250 ml hot water

1 Crush the caraway and fennel seeds in a mortar and pestle to help extract the oils. Combine the seeds with the peppermint and chamomile. Place in an airtight container.

2 To make the tea, put 1–2 tsp of the mix in 250 ml hot (not boiling) water and allow the herbs to infuse for about 15 minutes. Sip slowly, while still warm.

USE Drink a cup when required, up to 4 times a day.

STORAGE The herb mixture keeps very well in an airtight container for several months. Make the tea fresh before drinking.

Diarrhoea quickly drains the body of fluids, salts and other minerals. This recipe, which uses the World Health Organization formula for rehydration salts in the form of a stomach-soothing herbal tea, replaces electrolyte salts quickly and effectively. Take a tin of the salt and herb mixture with you whenever you're travelling.

DIARRHOEA
Herbal Rehydration Tea

½ tsp salt
¼ tsp potassium chloride ('low sodium' salt)
¼ tsp sodium bicarbonate
2 tbsp glucose
½–1 tbsp fennel seeds
½–1 tbsp peppermint leaves
1 litre water, boiled just before use

1 In a bowl, combine the salts, glucose and herbs, and mix well.

2 Add 1 litre of just boiled (though not boiling) water and allow the herbs to infuse for about 15 minutes. The seeds and leaves will sink to the bottom. Drink as much as possible to replace depleted electrolytes.

STORAGE The salt and herb mixture keeps very well in an airtight container for several months. Make the tea fresh before drinking.

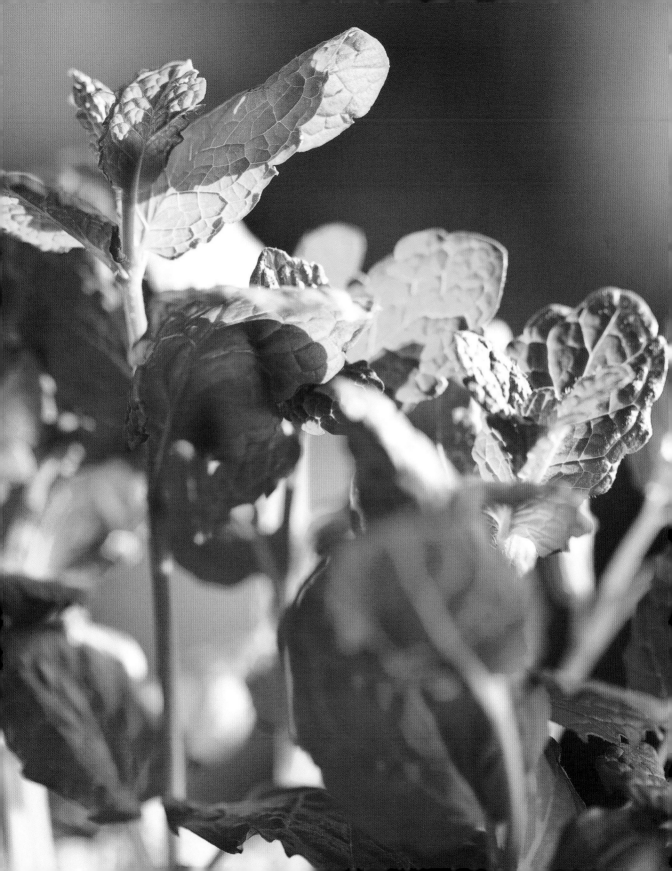

SKIN COMPLAINTS

Athlete's foot (*Tinea pedis*) is an irritating and sometimes painful fungal infection that thrives in the moist, dark areas between toes. This talc keeps feet dry, and the garlic and tea tree oil have potent anti-fungal properties. They help to beat foot odour, too. For a double hit, use in conjunction with the foot bath overleaf.

ATHLETE'S FOOT
Garlic Talcum Powder

4 tbsp dried sage leaves
4 tbsp dried garlic (commercially prepared is fine)
7 tbsp (70 g) cornflour
7 tbsp (70 g) bicarbonate of soda
24 drops tea tree oil

1 Grind the dried sage in a mortar and pestle, then place in a medium-sized bowl. Add the dried garlic. Sprinkle over the cornflour and bicarbonate of soda and mix well.

2 Add in the tea tree oil and stir until well distributed. Place the powder into a salt or sugar shaker for use.

USE Dust on liberally 3 times daily, until symptoms disappear (usually a few weeks). Continue using for 1 week after all signs of infection are gone, as previously dormant fungal spores can cause reinfection.
STORAGE Keep in a dry, dark place and use within 1 year.

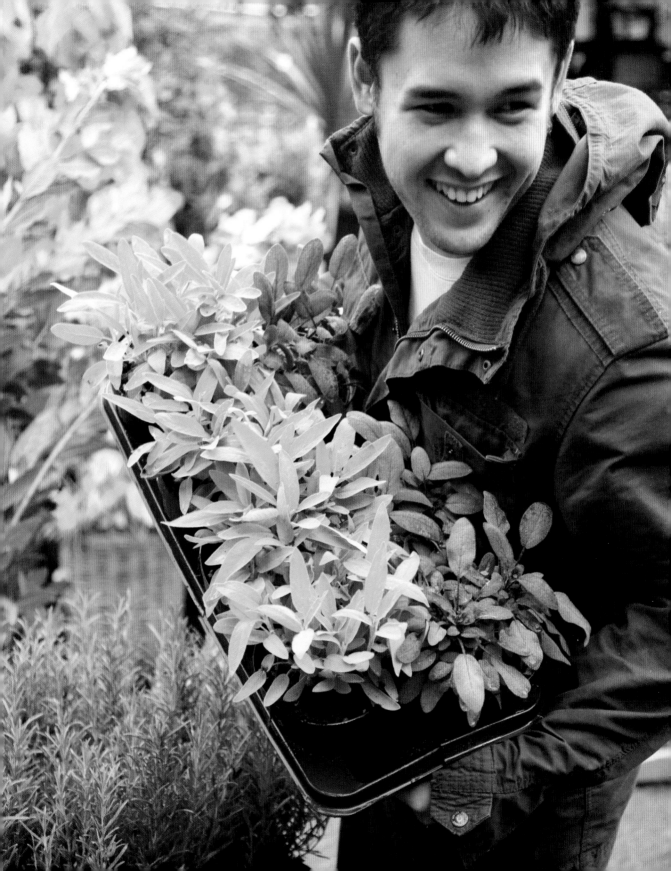

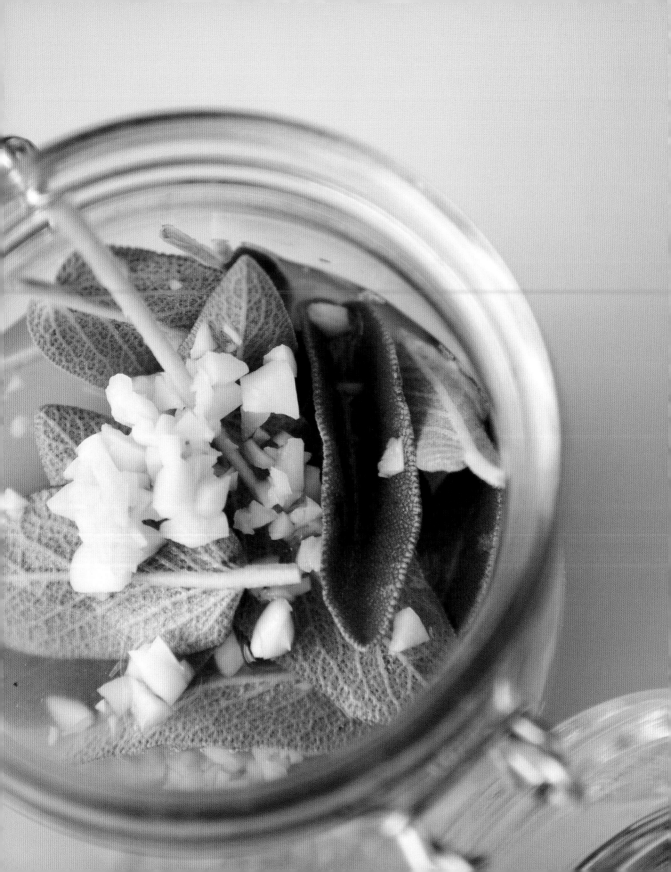

A few tablespoons of this garlicky vinegar in hot water make a powerful anti-fungal foot bath, but don't use it on broken skin – it will hurt! The vinegar takes 1 month to infuse, but will last at least 6 months and up to 1 year. It tastes good in salad dressings too.

ATHLETE'S FOOT

Garlic Foot Bath

10 bulbs garlic, finely chopped
100 g fresh sage leaves
500 ml cider vinegar

1 Place the chopped garlic and sage leaves in a jar, then add the cider vinegar. Seal and leave to infuse for 1 month, shaking occasionally.

USE Add 5 tbsp to a bowl of hot water, and soak feet for 15 minutes. Use 2–3 times a week in conjuction with Garlic Talcum Powder (see previous page).

The flowers of *Viola tricolor* have been used for centuries as an anti-inflammatory to treat skin conditions. Combined with the antihistamine and antiseptic properties of chamomile, it makes a soothing balm for eczema.

ECZEMA

Viola and Chamomile Cream

Makes one 150 ml pot
2 tbsp (20 g) viola flowers, stripped from their stems
2 tbsp (20 g) Roman or German chamomile, dried
250 ml freshly boiled water
1 tsp beeswax
2 tbsp almond oil
1 tsp vitamin C powder
1 tsp glycerine
2 tsp emulsifying wax

1 Place the violas and chamomile flowers in a glass bowl. Pour over the water to cover. Leave to infuse for 10 minutes. Put the infusion into a medium-sized pan (this will form the bottom of your double boiler or bain-marie).

2 In another glass bowl, add the beeswax, almond oil, vitamin C powder, glycerine and emulsifying wax. Place on top of the infusion pan, and warm over a gentle heat, stirring until melted. This takes about 10 minutes.

3 Strain the infusion, then slowly whisk it into the oil mixture until incorporated – the texture should be smooth, like mayonnaise.

4 Pour the mixture into a sterilized dark glass ointment pot, then seal.

USE Apply to affected areas morning and night. Ideally, apply within a few minutes of bathing, to keep moisture in the skin.
STORAGE Keeps for up to 6 months in the refrigerator.

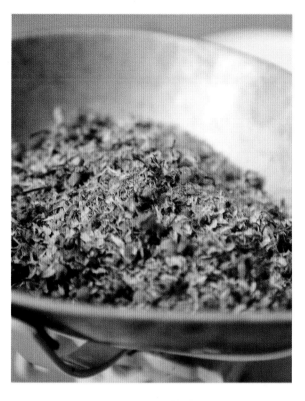

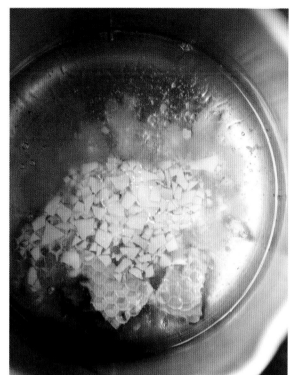

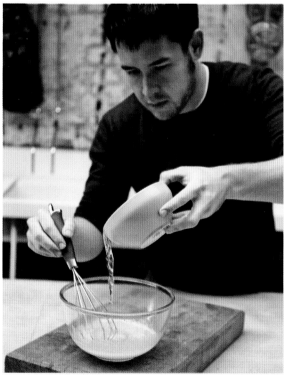

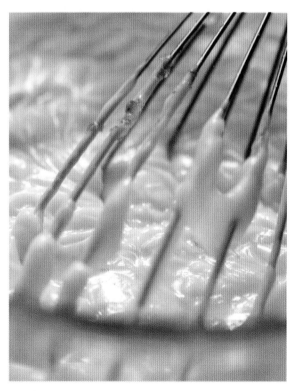

Insect bites cause immediate redness, swelling and itching. Take the heat out of them with plantain, which has both anti-inflammatory and anti-allergenic properties.

INSECT BITES AND STINGS

Plantain Cream

4 tbsp fresh plantain leaves
150 ml boiling water
2 tbsp olive oil or sunflower oil
2 tbsp almond oil
1 tsp beeswax
2 tsp emulsifying wax
2 tsp glycerine
1 tsp vitamin C powder

1 Wash and chop the plantain leaves. Divide into two – put one half in a bowl and the other half in a pan. Cover the plantain in the bowl with the water and leave to infuse for 10 minutes.

2 In the pan, add the olive (or sunflower) and almond oils to the plantain and heat gently to simmering point. Don't allow to boil – if it starts boiling, take off the heat immediately. Once at simmering point, remove from the heat and leave for 10 minutes to cool.

3 Drain the infusion, taking out the plantain leaves. Set the liquid to one side.

4 Drain the infused oil into another pan, extracting the plantain leaves. Heat the oil again. Add the beeswax and emulsifying wax and melt, stirring – you are aiming for a foamy consistency.

5 Add 16 tbsp infused water to the pan and whisk to achieve a consistency like salad dressing. Add the glycerine and vitamin C powder.

6 Pour into sterilized glass pots and seal.

USE Apply to affected area as often as needed.
STORAGE Keeps for 3 months in the refrigerator in an airtight container.

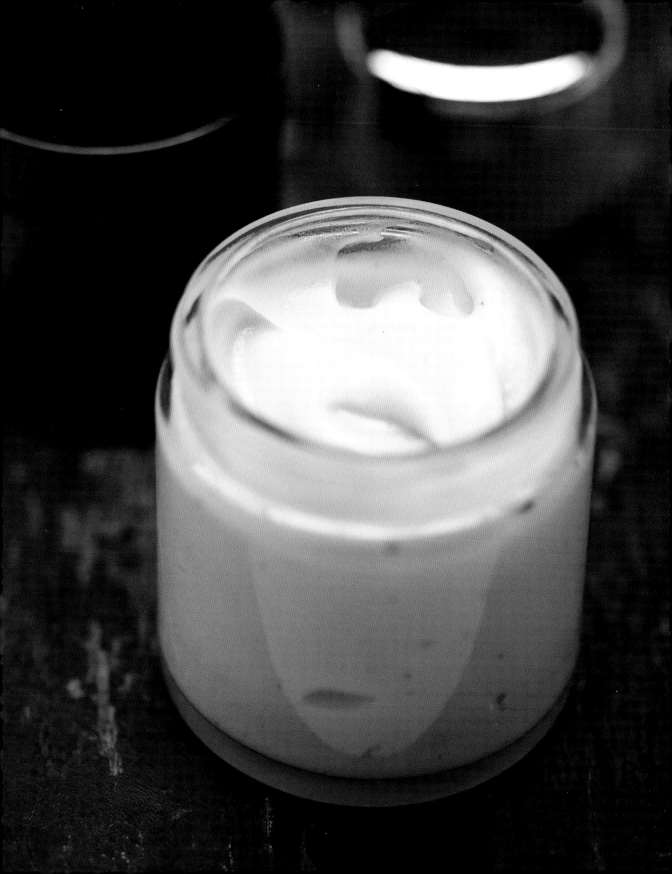

Native Americans traditionally used the leaves, bark and twigs of witch hazel (*Hamamelis virginiana*) as a skin compress. Its astringent, antibacterial properties make it especially useful for spots and pimples. This is gentler than many over-the-counter spot gels, which can leave skin dry and flaking. Carry a pot with you and dab on whenever needed.

SPOTS
Witch Hazel Gel

200 g witch hazel twigs and (preferably young) leaves
500 ml hot water
6 sachets vegetable gelatine
2 tbsp vodka

1 Place the witch hazel in a pan with the hot water. Over a gentle heat, slowly reduce to a third of its volume until you reach about 165 ml liquid (this will take about 1 hour).

2 Line a sieve with muslin, then strain the liquid through it into a mixing bowl. Add the gelatine, stirring to dissolve. Leave to cool.

3 Once cool, add the vodka and stir well, then pour the gel into a wide-mouthed jar.

USE Dab on spots and skin irritations whenever needed.
STORAGE Keeps for up to 6 months in the refrigerator.

The gel from the fleshy leaves of the aloe vera plant is excellent applied topically to soothe and speed the healing of sunburn and wounds. This gentle preparation can be used on children too.

SUNBURN

Carrot and Aloe Cream

2 carrots
1 cucumber
½ cup sesame oil
1 tsp beeswax
2 tsp emulsifying wax
½ cup aloe vera gel
1 tsp vitamin C powder

1 Finely grate the carrot and cucumber and place in a large pan with the sesame oil. Heat very gently for 20–30 minutes. Strain, then return the liquid to the pan.

2 Add the beeswax and emulsifying wax to the pan, and stir while they melt. Whisk in the aloe vera and vitamin C powder. Keep whisking until the mixture goes creamy and smooth.

3 Pour into a wide-mouthed jar, and leave to cool. The cream will thicken while cooling.

USE Apply liberally to any sunburnt or sore areas, 2–3 times a day.
STORAGE Keeps for up to 2 months in the refrigerator.

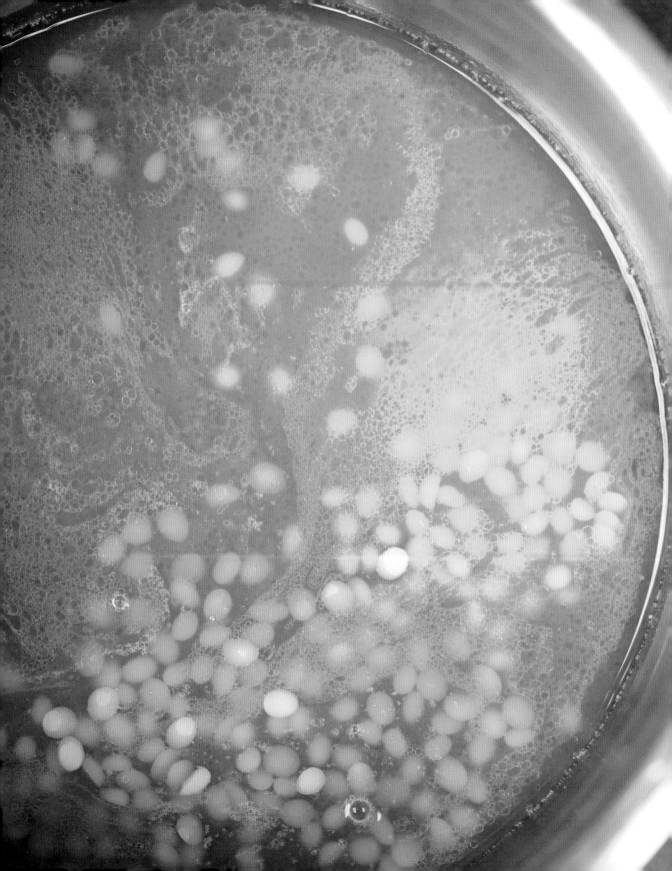

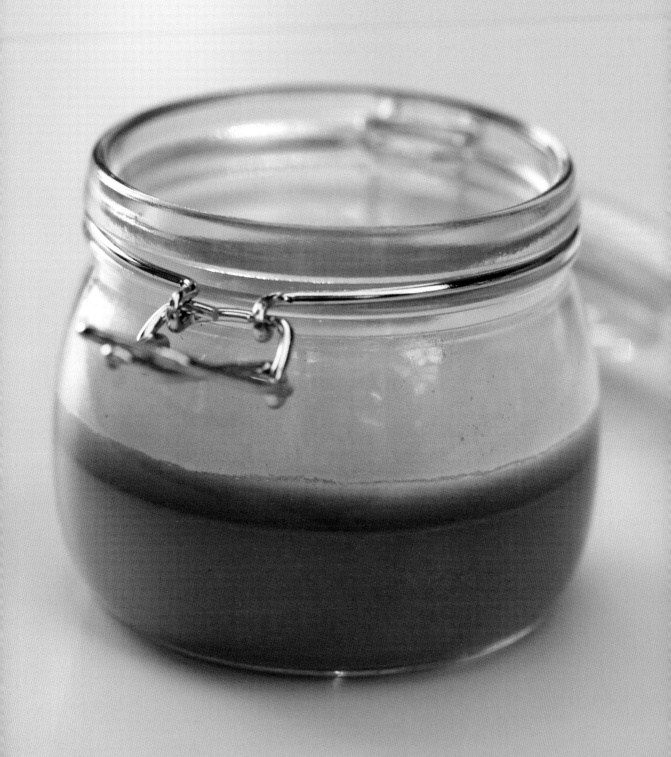

Bright orange pot marigold flowers (*Calendula officinalis*) contain salicylic acid – used in many over-the-counter acne treatments – plus anti-inflammatory and antiseptic substances, which make it a favourite for skin conditions of many kinds. Used over a period of weeks, this gel should significantly alleviate the appearance of acne and reduce discomfort.

ACNE

Marigold, Lavender and Rose Geranium Gel

10 rose geranium flowers, with leaves and stems
8 marigold (*Calendula officinalis*) flowers
20 lavender flowerheads
200 ml water
1 sachet vegetable gelatine
5 tsp vodka
20 drops tea tree oil

1 Roughly chop the flowers, leaves and stems of the rose geranium and place with the marigold flowers and lavender flowerheads in a large glass bowl.

2 Bring the water to the boil and pour it over the flowers to make an infusion. Leave to infuse for 10 minutes, or until the water has taken on the colour of the flowers. Place the infusion, including the plant material, into a blender and whiz. Strain the mixture through a piece of muslin into a clean bowl.

3 Now, in another bowl, dissolve the gelatine in 2 tbsp cold water. Gradually add the flower infusion, stirring to separate lumps. Add the vodka and tea tree oil, stirring until a gel is formed. Using a funnel, pour into a pot with a pump dispenser.

USE Apply to affected areas 2 times a day, or as frequently as needed.
STORAGE Keeps in the refrigerator for up to 6 weeks.

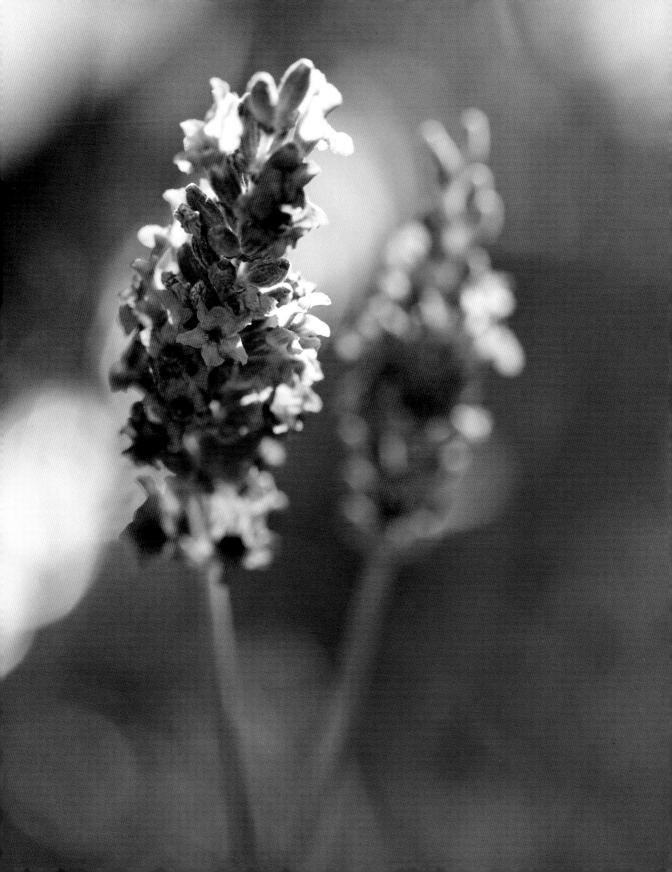

This is excellent for ringworm, athlete's foot and thrush.
It is also makes a good antiseptic hand wash because both
tea tree and thyme are potent anti-fungals. Soap moulds
can be bought online.

FUNGAL SKIN CONDITIONS

Antiseptic Soap

300 g white soap
500 ml water
5 tbsp almond oil (or olive, jojoba or avocado oil)
2 tsp tea tree essential oil
30 drops thyme (*Thymus vulgaris,* ct. linalool) essential oil
4 tbsp dried marigold (*Calendula officinalis*) flowers

1 Grate the white soap into a glass bowl, then add the water. Place the bowl over a pan of boiling water on a low heat. Stir continuously until the soap melts.

2 Add the almond oil, and tea tree and thyme essential oils. Throw in the dried flowers, mixing well with a metal spoon.

3 Pour the mixture into a shallow dish to make a soap 'loaf', or into individual soap moulds. Leave to cool and set; this might take up to 1 week.

4 Once set, cut the soap loaf into shapes or turn out of the moulds. Wrap the soaps in greaseproof paper and leave to dry in a cool place until needed.

USE Wash affected areas with the soap once or twice daily, or as required. Rinse off well.
STORAGE Store, wrapped in greaseproof paper, in a cool, dark place. Keeps for up to 1 year.

Juniper (*Juniperus communis*) contains powerful anti-inflammatory and astringent substances. Use the oil in massage to stimulate circulation and relieve back pain, and the healing ointment to soothe burn scars, itching and scratches.

HEALING OINTMENT
Juniper Oil

125 g fresh juniper berries (preferably just ripening)
250 ml olive or sunflower oil
3–4 tbsp beeswax (for ointment only)

To make the massage oil:

1 Soak the berries in water overnight to soften, then strain and discard the water.

2 Place the berries in a double boiler or bain-marie, then add the oil and simmer gently, taking care not to burn, for 30 minutes, or until the berries lose their colour and the oil darkens.

3 Strain through a sieve lined with muslin, reserving the oil. Pour into a sterilized glass bottle to store.

USE Massage well into the affected area 2–3 times a day.
STORAGE Keeps for at least 6 months.

To make the healing ointment:

Make the Juniper Oil as described. Heat the beeswax in a double boiler or bain-marie over a low heat. Stir in the oil, mixing thoroughly. Pour into a sterilized dark glass jar. As it cools the balm will solidify. If the ointment is too soft, remove from the pot and add a little more melted wax. Gently reheat the mixture until smooth, then bottle as before.

USE Apply 2–3 times a day to scar or affected area.
STORAGE Keeps for 6 months in a sterilized dark glass jar.

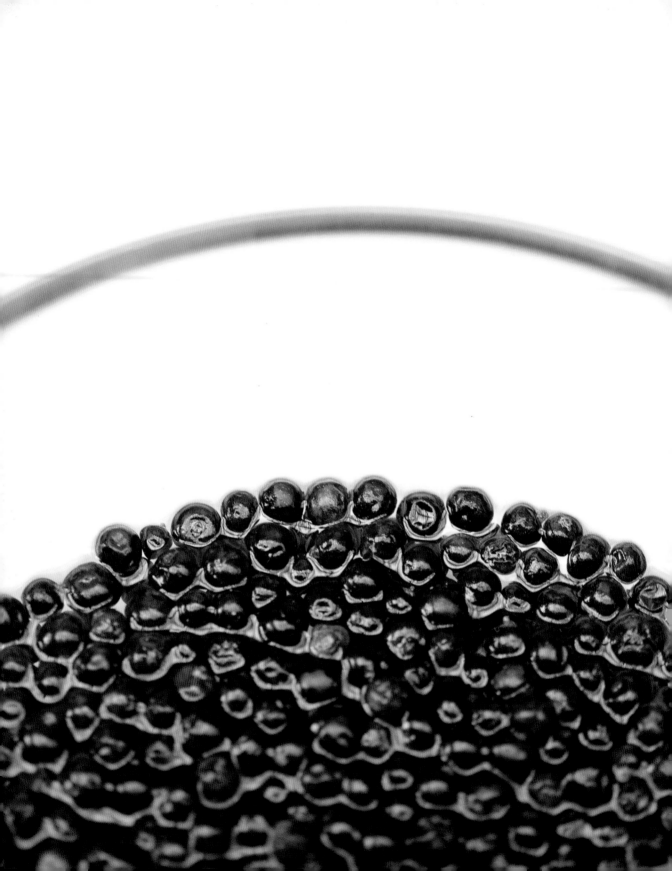

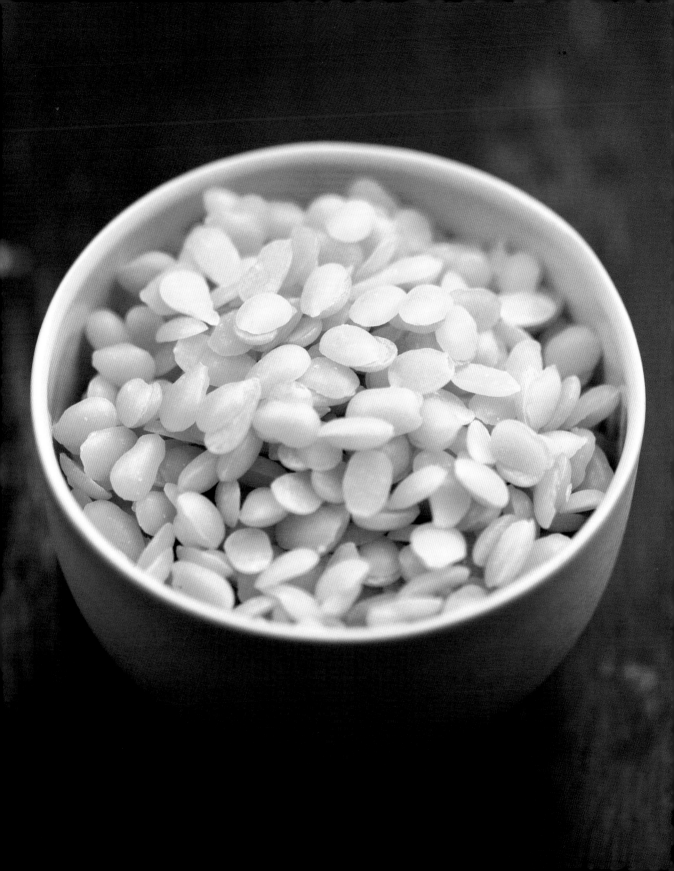

This makes the blood race to your feet. Apply every day before bed to improve circulation and help prevent cold feet and chilblains.

COLD FEET
Hot Chilli and Mustard Foot Oil

500 ml sunflower oil
2–4 fresh whole red chillis (cayenne), chopped
50 g ginger root, chopped or crushed
50 g black pepper
50 g mustard powder

1 In a bain-marie or glass bowl (to form the top of a double boiler), place the sunflower oil, chopped chillis, ginger, black pepper and mustard powder. Stir to mix. Place the bowl, covered, on a pan of hot water, and heat the mixture gently for 1 hour.

2 Strain through a sieve lined with muslin. Filter the oil into sterilized dark glass bottles.

USE Rub a little directly into the feet at night to encourage circulation.
NB This oil does heat the skin, so wash your hands after use and keep away from eyes and other sensitive areas.
STORAGE Keeps for up to 6 months.

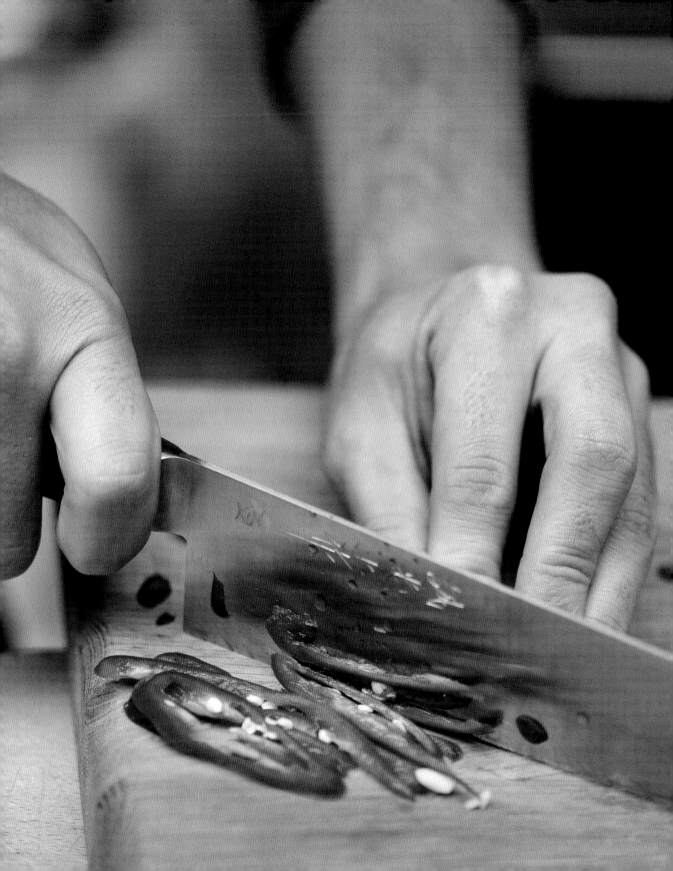

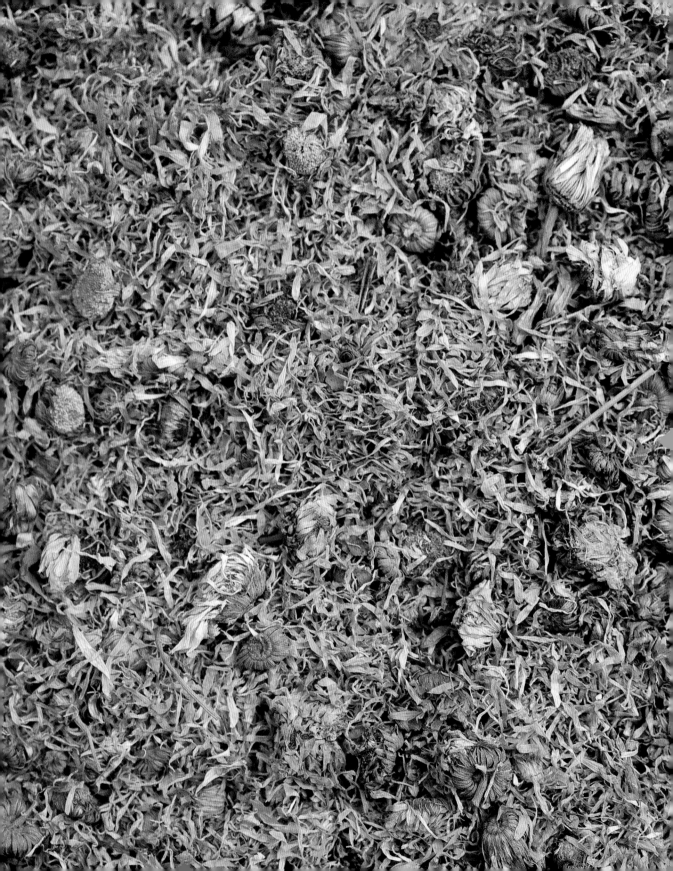

This gentle salve for chapped hands, skin inflammations, wounds and piles is very easy to make. Eucalyptus has a powerful aroma that you either love or hate – leave it out if you wish.

CHAPPED HANDS AND SORES

Jelly Balm

25 g St John's wort flowers
20 g marigold (*Calendula officinalis*) flowers
olive oil, to cover
white petroleum jelly – 2 parts to 1 part of oil
eucalpytus oil (optional)

1 Put the St John's wort and marigold flowers in a jar and cover with the olive oil. Allow to stand in a cool place for 1 week and then strain through muslin.

2 Melt the petroleum jelly in a double boiler or bain-marie. Add 1 part of the oil made above to 2 parts of melted petroleum jelly. Stir while cooling – you can also add a few drops of eucalyptus oil at this stage if you like. Pour into a sterilized glass jar before the ointment solidifies.

USE Gently rub into the affected area 3–4 times a day when needed.
STORAGE Keeps for at least 6 months in a refrigerator.

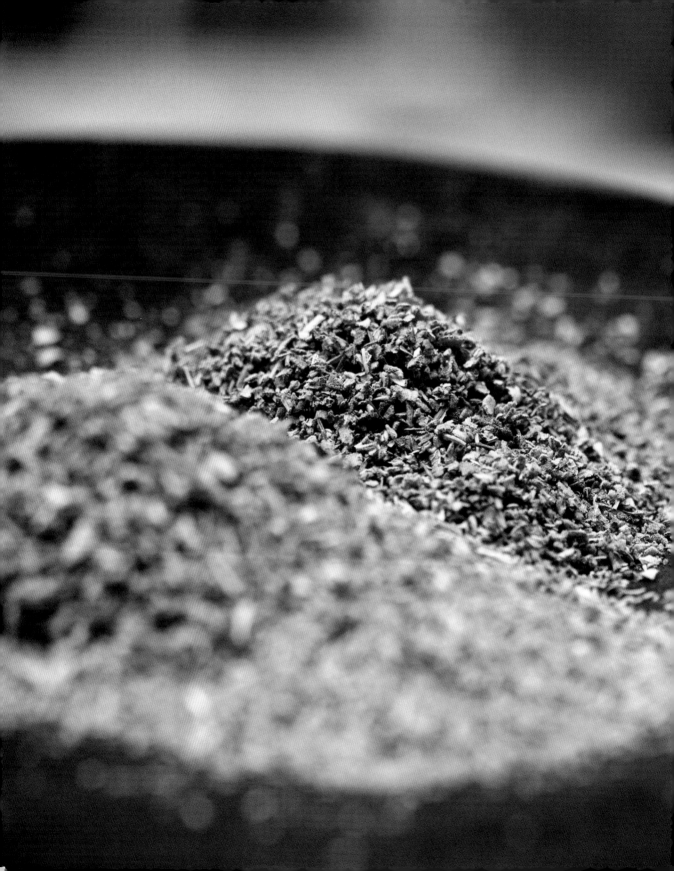

This is a very simple way to deter flying pests and protect yourself from bites and stings. Sage, rosemary and wormwood are well known as insect repellents, containing camphor and other essential oils. You can use bought dried herbs, though drying your own from fresh will produce a more aromatic mix.

INSECT DETERRENT
Pest Pot-Pourri

2 tbsp dried rosemary leaves
2 tbsp dried wormwood leaves
2 tbsp dried sage leaves

Strip the leaves from the plants, and crush them finely. Mix together in an open shallow bowl, and leave in a warm place in the room to encourage the oils to vaporize.

STORAGE Keeps for at least 1 month, or until the aroma has gone.

KIDS

An old-fashioned winter remedy for boosting vitamin levels and keeping colds at bay. Gather the hips in October and November when they're ripe and soft. Children love this syrup, and it's good poured over pancakes, waffles, ice-cream and rice pudding.

VITAMIN BOOSTER
Vitamin C-rich Rosehip Syrup

250 g fresh rosehips
5 cloves (optional)
1 cinnamon stick (optional)
500 ml water
about 125 g sugar

1 Crush the rosehips slightly, and place in a pan. Add the cloves and cinnamon stick, if using, then add the water. Simmer, uncovered, for 20 minutes.

2 Strain, then add the same amount of sugar as there is liquid (about 125 g). Stir until dissolved and bring to the boil, then simmer for 10 minutes. Cool and filter into small, sterilized bottles.

USE For children, give 2 tsp per day; dilute 1 part syrup to 5 parts water and drink as a cordial; or use instead of maple syrup for the dishes suggested above.
STORAGE Keeps for 1 week in the refrigerator once opened. Unopened, Keeps for up to 1 year.

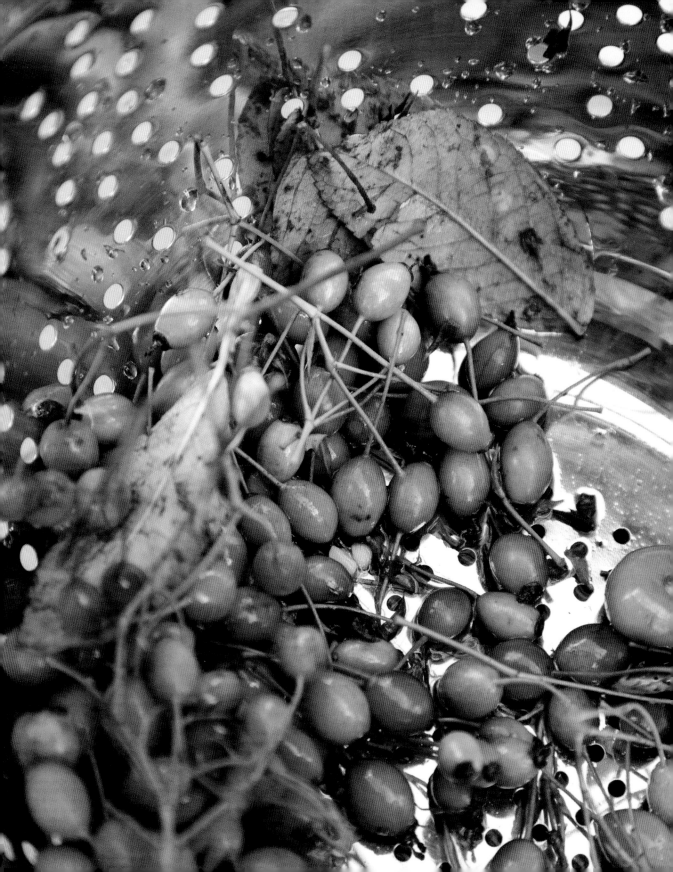

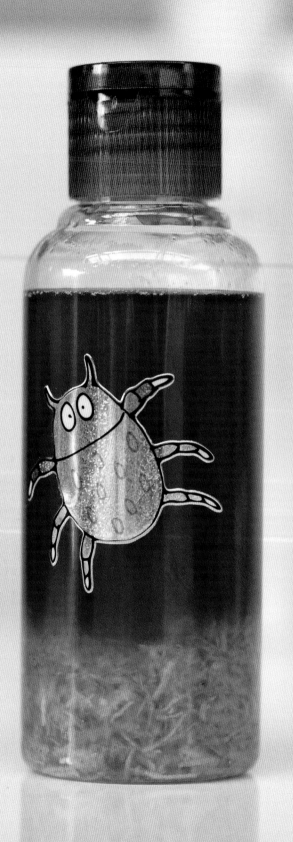

With up to 80% of head lice now resistant to conventional treatments, the hunt is on for an effective and safe insecticide to treat nits. This natural recipe, free of organophosphates, uses plant extracts with known insecticidal properties to kill both lice and the nits – the tiny eggs that are notoriously hard to eradicate.

HEAD LICE
Neem Nit Treatment

Makes enough for 5–10 doses
20 tbsp (approx. 100 g) fresh rosemary leaves
20 tbsp (approx. 25 g) fresh lavender flowers
200 ml neem oil
200 ml almond oil
6 garlic cloves, minced
2 tbsp tea tree oil

1 Strip the rosemary leaves and lavender flowers from their sprigs.

2 Combine the neem and almond oil together in a measuring jug.

3 Crush half the rosemary and lavender in a mortar and pestle with a little of the oil, to help ease the crushing process. Place the mashed-up herbs in a saucepan. Repeat with the second half of the rosemary and lavender, again adding a little oil for crushing.

4 Place the crushed herbs, neem and almond oil in the pan, and add the chopped garlic. Heat gently for about 20 minutes.

5 Strain through a sieve lined with muslin. Add the tea tree oil to the reserved oil, stir, then filter into a sterilized 500 ml bottle.

USE If using immediately, apply to dry hair, making sure that the hair is completely covered and that the oil penetrates to the scalp. Cover with a towel and leave on for at least 1 hour, or overnight if possible. Then wash off with two applications of shampoo. Apply conditioner, and comb through with a nit comb. Use the next application 7 days later, to deal with any nits that may hatch during that time. Comb through with the nit comb every 3 days.
STORAGE Keeps for 6 months.

A wonderful way to give herbs to children is simply by adding them to the bath. This infusion – made with Roman instead of German chamomile – soothes eczema, the red, itchy, inflamed skin condition that is extremely common in children and babies. The flowerheads bob around like pom-poms and are fun for children to play with.

ECZEMA

Pom-pom Bath

4 handfuls (approx. 40 g) Roman chamomile
  (*Chamaemelum nobile*) flowerheads
1 litre freshly boiled water

Place the chamomile in a glass bowl, then add 1 litre of freshly boiled water and leave, covered, for about 15 minutes.

USE Add straight to bath water. Alternatively, strain the flowerheads out.
STORAGE Make fresh before use.

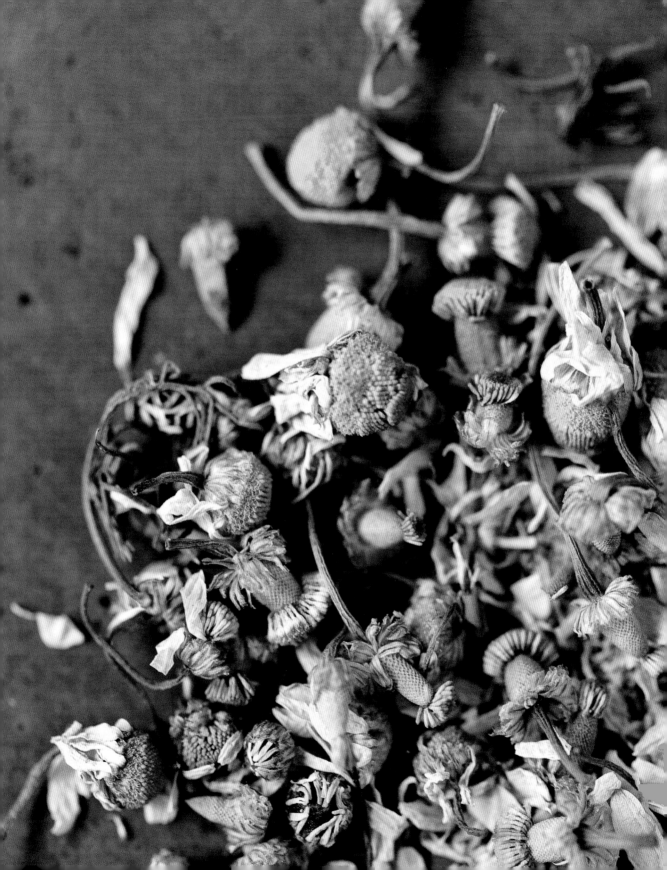

A simple remedy containing mullein (*Verbascum thapsus*), traditionally used to soothe inflammation and aid healing, and almond oil to soften wax.

EAR WAX BUILD-UP
Wax-dissolving Drops

1 small handful mullein flowers
250 ml almond oil

1 Cover the mullein flowers with the oil, and steep for several days in sunlight.

2 Alternatively, you can place the flowers and oil in a small pan and warm on the stove on a very gentle heat for several hours.

3 Strain through muslin and a small filter into sterilized dropper bottles.

USE Instil a few drops into the affected ear(s) morning and night, or up to 4 times a day to relieve pain and soften wax. Continue treatment for at least 5 days.
NB If the wax is very hard, the ear may need syringing by your GP. These drops will make that process easier.
STORAGE Keeps for 3 months.

Sweet syrups are an easy way to get children to take herbal remedies. This multi-tasking chamomile syrup has a calming, sedative effect, relaxes the digestive tract, and has anti-allergenic properties. Good for use with colic, tummy aches, and when a child has trouble sleeping.

COLIC

Chamomile Syrup

40 g German chamomile (*Matricaria recutita*) flowerheads
900 ml water
450 g sugar or honey

1 In a pan, put the chamomile in the water and bring to the boil. Turn the heat to low, then cover with a tight-fitting lid and simmer for about 20 minutes.

2 Reduce the mixture to 200 ml, by simmering very slowly with the lid off for a further 20 minutes.

3 Add the sugar, and simmer for a few more minutes, stirring all the time until the mixture looks like syrup. Be careful not to boil rapidly; allow it to bubble just a little.

4 Strain through a mesh sieve and pour it into a sterilized bottle. Seal with a cork; if the syrup ferments, the bottle might explode.

USE For a child, 1 tsp, 3–6 times a day. For adults, 2–4 tsp, 3–6 times daily. NB Not to be used by diabetics.
STORAGE Keeps unopened for up to 1 year. Once opened, keep for 1 week in the refrigerator.

ACHES AND PAINS

Swollen ankles, feet and lower legs often get more painful as the day progresses. Plantain, dandelion and nettle, probably the three most common garden weeds, are all mild diuretics and are traditionally used to ease the symptoms caused by water retention. The dandelion restores potassium levels, which can be flushed out by many diuretics.

WATER RETENTION
Plantain Tea for Swollen Ankles

2 tbsp fresh plantain leaves
2 tbsp fresh dandelion leaves (or flowers)
2 tbsp nettle leaves
1 litre water, freshly boiled

Wash the leaves, place in a bowl, then pour over the water. Steep for 10 minutes. Strain.

USE This makes enough for about 3 cups, to be drunk throughout the day.

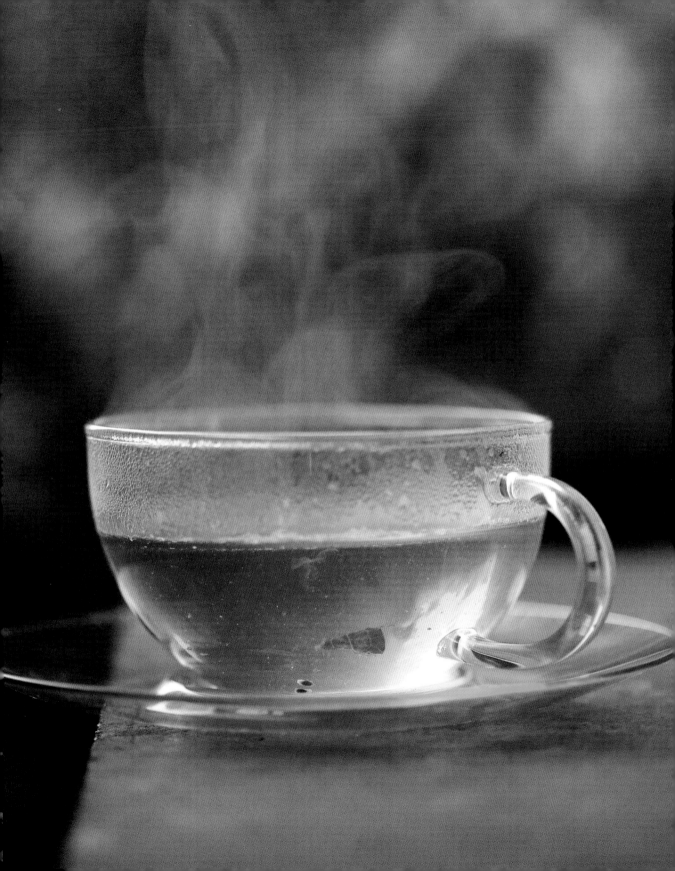

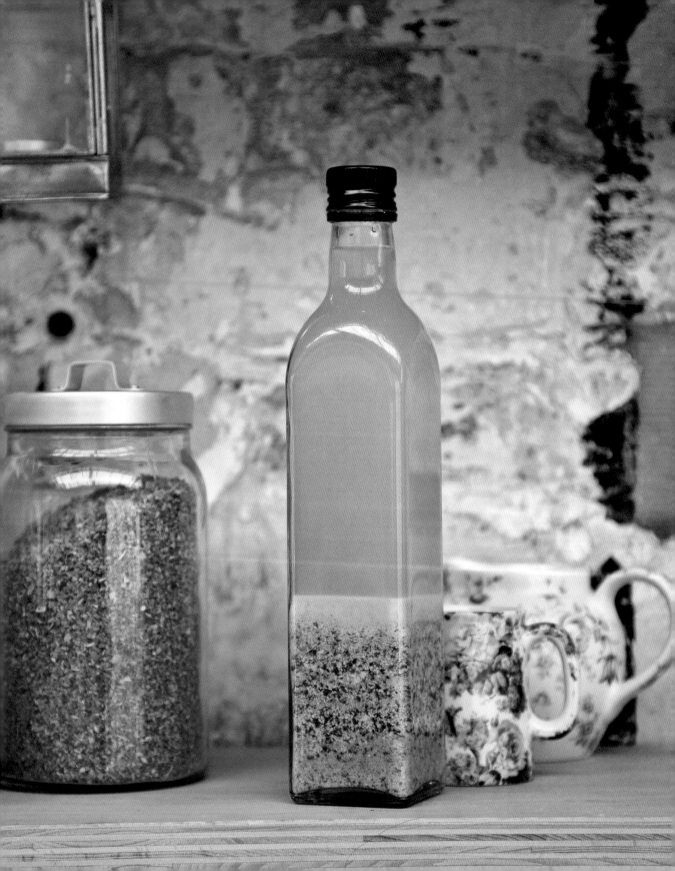

You can pick up conkers (the seeds of *Aesculus hippocastanum*) by the basketload in autumn. They contain saponins, which are frequently used in the treatment of varicose veins (and piles) to improve the elasticity of the walls of the veins, reducing swelling and relieving the feeling of heaviness in the legs. Prepare the tincture first, then use to make the gel (see overleaf).

VARICOSE VEIN GEL
Horse Chestnut Tincture

20 conkers
500 ml vodka

1 Blend the conkers and vodka in a liquidizer until smooth.

2 Place in a sterilized bottle and keep in a cool dark place for 10 days to 1 month, shaking every day or so. Strain before using.

STORAGE Keeps for up to 1 year.
NB This tincture is only to be used to make the Horse Chestnut Gel (see overleaf), and must not be taken internally.

This slightly astringent gel feels cool and refreshing on sore, swollen legs and varicose veins. Can be used on long flights to reduce swelling.

VARICOSE VEINS
Horse Chestnut Gel

3 sachets vegetable gelatine
150 ml water
150 ml Horse Chestnut Tincture (see page 87)
5 drops lavender oil

1 Add the vegetable gelatine to 150 ml cold water in a pan and whisk until dissolved. Heat for about 2 minutes, whisking constantly. As the mix starts to thicken, slowly pour in the Horse Chestnut Tincture a little at a time. Add the lavender oil.

2 Pour into a 250 ml sterilized bottle.

USE Try a 24-hour patch test before using — horse chestnut can irritate. Apply to affected areas twice daily, or as often as required.
STORAGE The gel keeps for 3 months in the refrigerator.

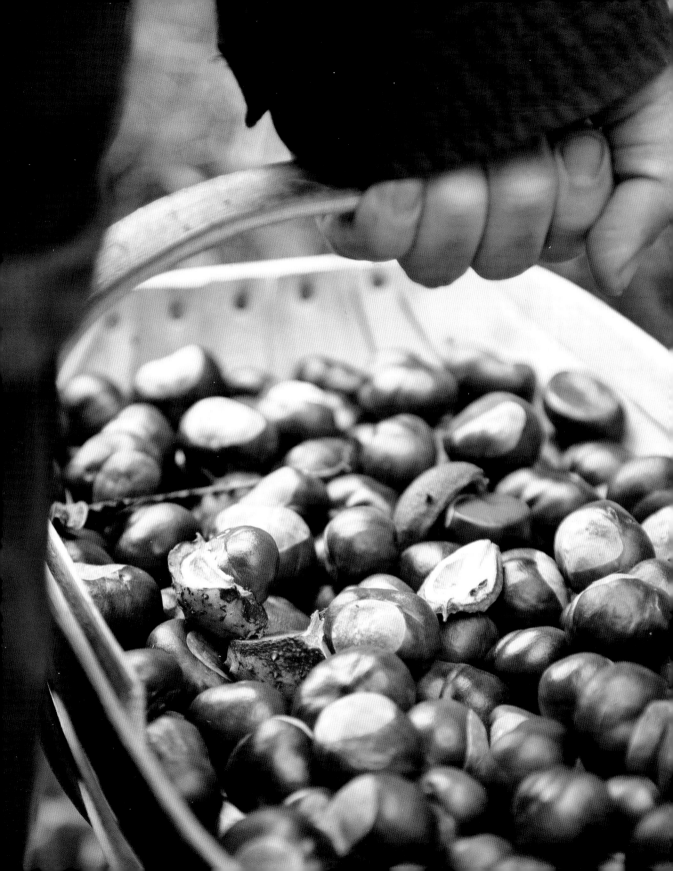

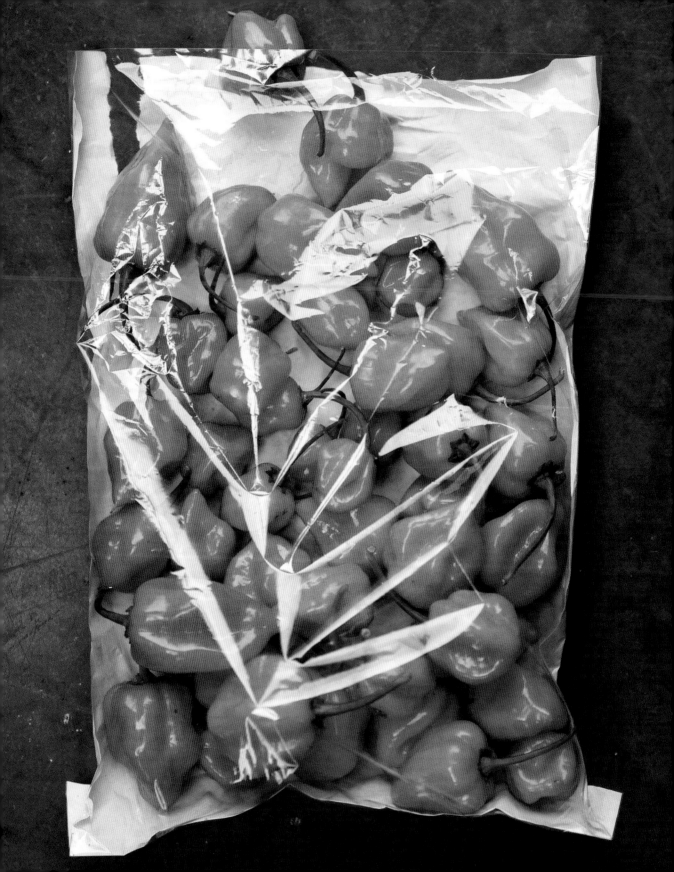

Chilli and mustard work as both a local anaesthetic and a deep-heat treatment to ease stiff and painful muscles. This makes 4–5 plasters. Non-fractionated coconut oil is available in ethnic food stores. It should be white and solid at room temperature.

FOR ACHING MUSCLES
Chilli Plasters

200 g orange Scotch Bonnet chillies
4 tbsp mustard powder
200 g coconut oil, non-fractionated
6 tsp beeswax
4 packs Melolin wound dressing pads, 10 x 10 cm
4 packs adhesive wound dressing, 12 x 12 cm

1 Wash and finely slice the chillies. Combine the chillies and mustard powder with the coconut oil in a saucepan. Cover to keep in the vapour and gently heat for 2 minutes. Leave to cool with the lid on.

2 Put the chilli mix into muslin over a sieve and squeeze out the oil into a bowl below. Place the oil back into the saucepan and return to the heat.

3 Add the beeswax to the oil and heat very gently until dissolved; this will take less than 2 minutes. Remove from the heat.

4 Soak the dressing pads in the oil mixture while it's still hot. When they are saturated, remove the pads and leave to stand for 10 minutes on greaseproof paper, or until set.

5 Once set and dry, the pads can be layered on top of each other, wrapped in clingfilm and stored in the refrigerator until needed.

USE Place a pad on an adhesive wound dressing, then apply to the affected area. Keep the area warm (by covering with a blanket, for example) and leave on for 30 minutes to 1 hour.
STORAGE Keeps for 1 year in the refrigerator.

VARIATION
Chilli Talcum Powder

Both chilli powder and mustard powder can be used to make a warming 'talc' that invigorates circulation. Mix together 1 tsp chilli powder, 1 tsp mustard power and 1 tbsp cornflour, and use this to dust cold feet with before putting socks on.

To soothe the pain of both hot and cold arthritic joints, try this spicy remedy, countered with peppermint and rosemary oils for scent and pain relief.

ARTHRITIS

Chilli and Peppermint Salve

60 ml Hot Chilli and Mustard Foot Oil
(see page 70)
20 g beeswax
30 drops peppermint essential oil
30 drops rosemary essential oil

1 Put the oil in a glass bowl (to use as the top of a double boiler) or bain-marie. Add the beeswax. Place over a pan of hot water and heat gently, stirring occasionally, until the wax melts. Take off the heat and allow to cool.

2 Just as a 'skin' begins to appear on the surface of the oils, add the peppermint and rosemary oils using a dropper. Mix well. Pour the mixture into a sterilized dark glass jar. Allow to cool before putting on the lid.

USE Apply twice daily to affected areas, remembering to wash hands after use. NB This oil is hot, so keep away from eyes and other sensitive areas.
STORAGE Keeps for up to 6 months.

VARIATION
Cabbage Leaf Poultice

1 Cabbage leaf has been used for centuries for swellings, ulcers, sprains and strains. In one Swiss hospital, patients with rheumatoid arthritis have their swollen joints wrapped up at night in cabbage leaves to help reduce joint swelling and pain.

2 Savoy cabbages work best: take some cabbage leaves, cut out the central rib, lay them flat on a chopping board and bash with a rolling pin until the juices start to come out. Then place the leaves over swollen joints, and wrap round with a crêpe bandage to keep the leaves in place.

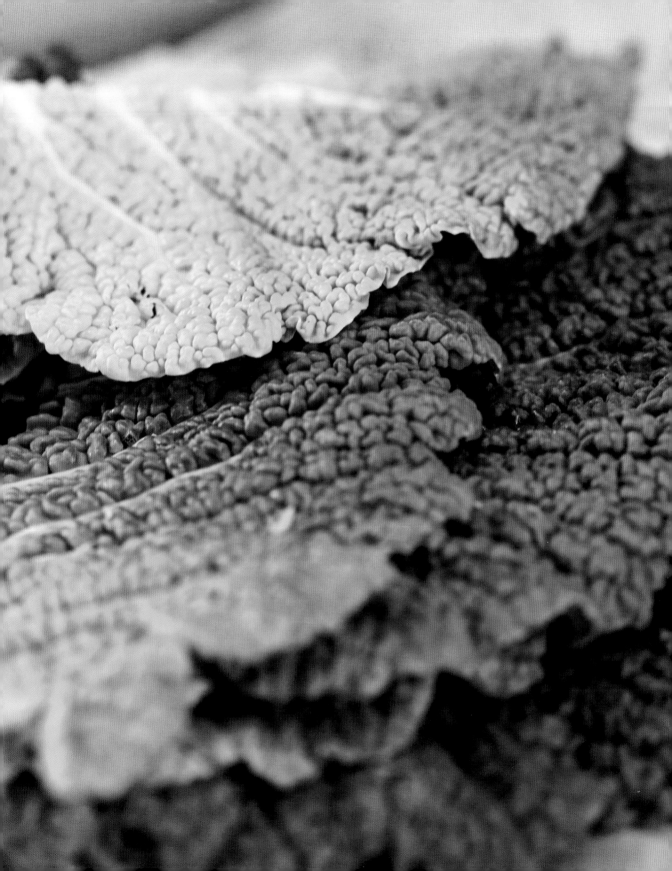

WOMEN'S STUFF

Try this simple tea for hot flushes and night sweats. No one quite knows why sage reduces sweating – possibly because of its astringency – while raspberry leaves are traditionally used to balance female hormones. Make this tea up fresh before drinking.

HOT FLUSHES AND NIGHT SWEATS
Sage and Raspberry Leaf Tea

½ tbsp fresh sage leaves
   (if dried, use half the amount)
½ tbsp fresh raspberry leaves
   (if dried, use half the amount)
200 ml freshly boiled water

Pour the water over the washed sage and raspberry leaves, and leave to infuse for 8–10 minutes.

USE Sip a small wine glassful every 3 hours. NB Not to be used by pregnant women.

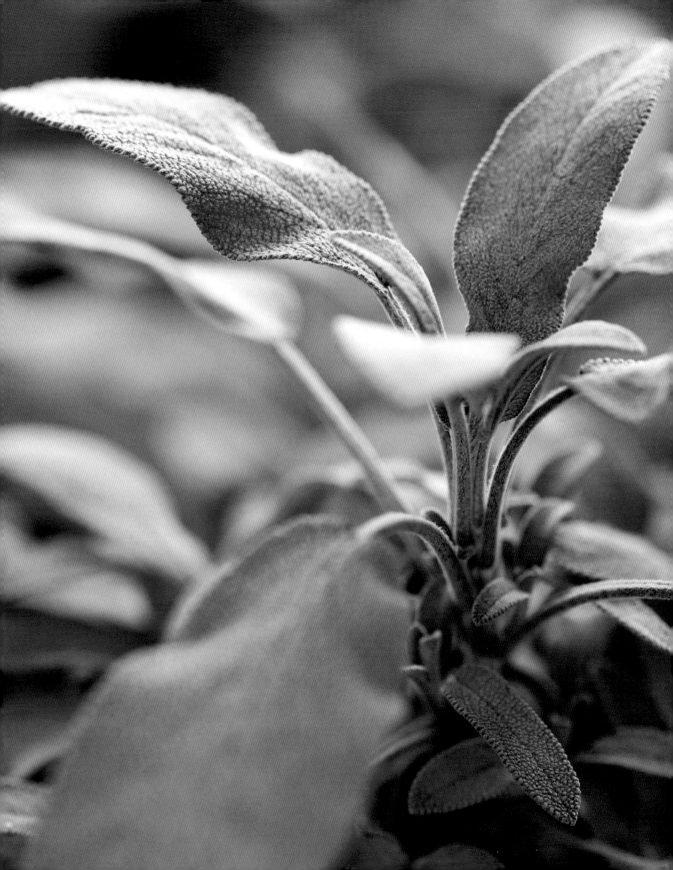

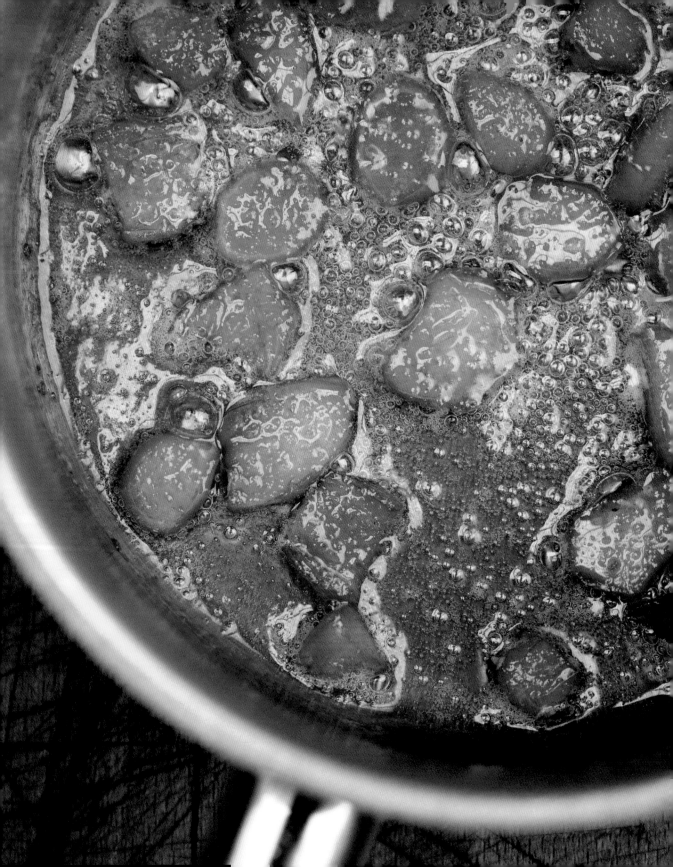

Ginger is a safe and effective treatment for both morning and travel sickness. These slices of crystallized ginger are easy to keep in a small jar in your handbag or desk, and great to chew on when you're feeling queasy.

MORNING AND TRAVEL SICKNESS

Crystallized Ginger

Makes about 250 g
350 g fresh ginger root
golden caster sugar, to match weight of cooked ginger,
    plus extra for sprinkling

1 Peel the fresh ginger root and thinly slice.

2 Put the ginger in a heavy-bottomed saucepan and cover with water, adding more to allow for evaporation. Bring to the boil and partly cover with a lid. Boil gently for 1 hour, or until the ginger is almost cooked but slightly al dente; the time will vary slightly depending on the freshness of ginger.

3 Drain the ginger and weigh it. Put it back in the saucepan with an equal amount of golden caster sugar. Add 2 tbsp water. Bring to the boil, then simmer over a medium heat, stirring with a wooden spoon for 20 minutes, or until it starts to go gloopy and the ginger becomes transparent.

4 Reduce the heat and keep stirring until it starts to crystallize and easily piles up in the middle of the pan.

5 Meanwhile take a large, deep, baking tray and sprinkle caster sugar on it. Tip the ginger into the baking tray and shuffle it round in the caster sugar. Separate any clumps of ginger pieces. Place in a sterilized jar.

USE Chew on a piece of crystallized ginger when you feel nauseous.
STORAGE Keeps in a cool place for 3–6 months.

VARIATION
Ginger Tea
For an easy anti-nausea tea, peel and roughly slice a 2 cm piece of root ginger into a cup, and pour over boiling water. Add 1 tsp honey to sweeten, if preferred, and a slice of lemon. Leave to infuse for a few minutes, then drink.

Browny-black chaste berries (*Vitex agnus-castus*) contain remarkable hormone-regulating substances, which have been shown to be effective in alleviating symptoms of premenstrual syndrome (PMS). This vinegar can help to minimize the backache, stomach cramps, breast tenderness, irritability and mood swings that arrive as part of the monthly cycle.

PMS

Chaste Berry Vinegar

200 ml good-quality cider vinegar
50 g chaste berries, fresh or dried

Pour the vinegar over the berries in a jar. Seal. Shake every day for 2 weeks. Strain, and return to the jar.

USE Take 1 tsp every day.
NB Not to be used during pregnancy.
STORAGE Keeps for 6 months in a dark place.

Snack on this chewy dried fruit treat regularly to prevent cystitis. It is equally effective if you're suffering an acute attack. Cranberry works by preventing bacteria from attaching to the wall of the bladder, where they start multiplying. This fruit leather is easy to carry round, so keep some in your desk or handbag for use every day.

CYSTITIS

Cranberry Fruit Leather

500 g fresh, ripe cranberries
caster sugar, to taste

1 Rinse the cranberries, then dry. Crush with a rolling pin to make a mash, collecting all the juice you can. Alternatively, if you prefer a smoother texture, whiz in a blender until puréed.

2 Line a baking tray with greaseproof parchment or baking paper. Press the berry mash into the tray, to a thickness of about 1 cm. Smooth the top. Place in the oven at the lowest setting (about 40–50°C), and leave for up to 12 hours. Keep checking to make sure the fruit does not overdry – you want a texture that holds its shape when pulled away from the parchment, but which does not crack or crumble.

3 Sprinkle over as little sugar as you can to make the fruit leather palatable. Leave the sugared leather in its tray to dry out for another 12 hours, or until it is completely dry.

4 Warm the leather in a very low oven for 10 minutes, then roll it and cut into slices. Store in an airtight container on greaseproof paper.

USE Chew on a strip as often as you like.
STORAGE Keeps in the refrigerator for about 1 month.

UNDER THE WEATHER

Echinacea lessens the severity and duration of colds and flu. Keep these ice lollies in the freezer to take when you feel the first signs of infection coming on.

COLDS AND FLU

Echinacea Ice Lollies

To make the tincture:
20 g fresh echinacea root
80 ml vodka

For the ice lollies:
2 medium-sized red chillis
8 cm root ginger
240 ml honey
1 sachet animal gelatine
800 ml cranberry juice
juice of 2 large lemons

80 ml Echinacea Tincture (see above)

1 Wash and chop the echinacea root, then put in a jar and pour over the vodka to cover completely. Leave for 2–4 weeks.

2 Wash and slice the chillis. Peel and thinly slice the ginger.

3 Combine the chillis, ginger, honey, gelatine and cranberry juice in a saucepan, then stir and simmer for 5 minutes. Take off the heat and leave to cool. Sieve into a bowl.

4 When the drained liquid is cool, stir in the lemon juice and Echinacea Tincture. Pour into ice lolly moulds and freeze.

USE Take during colds or infection.
NB Contains alcohol.
STORAGE The lollies keep in the freezer for 3 months.

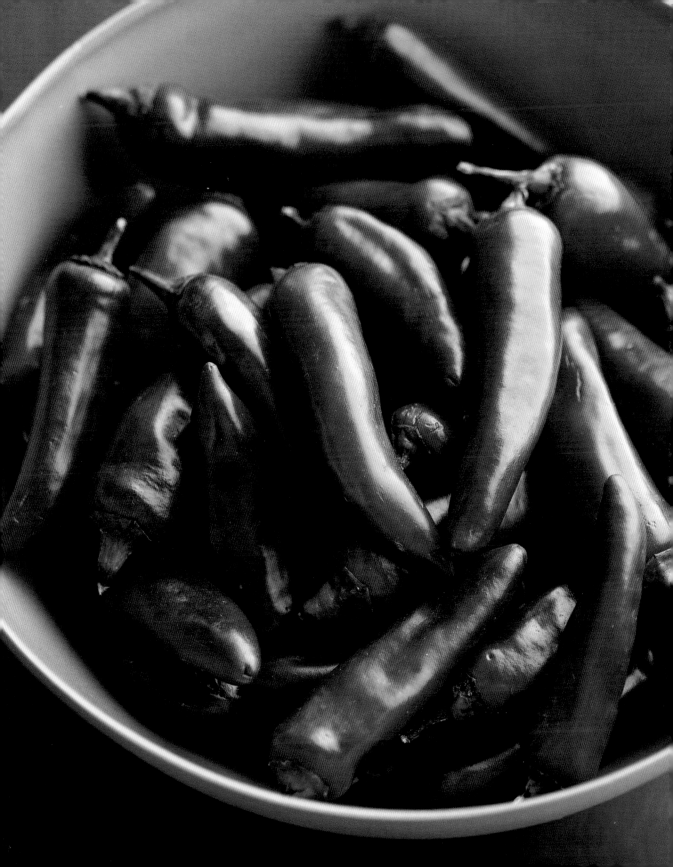

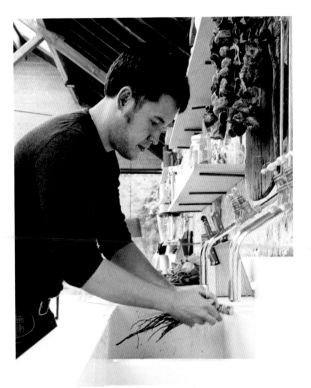

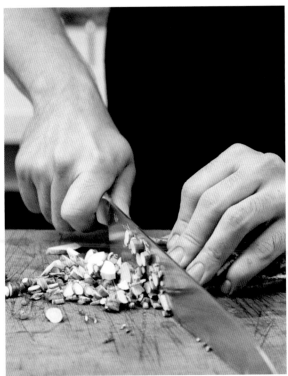

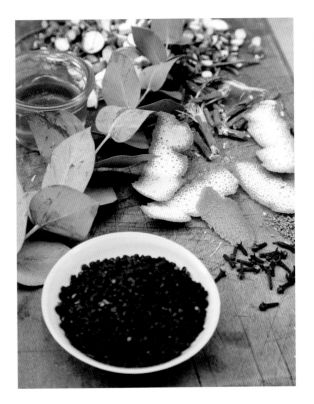

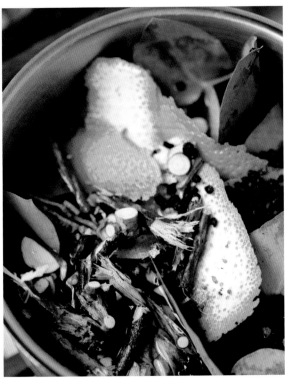

Liquorice has been used for centuries as an expectorant to loosen phlegm. When mixed with marshmallow, which contains a soothing mucilage, it reduces coughing and help soothe sore throats. This syrup is especially good for dry or tickly coughs. Quantities differ depending on whether you use fresh or dried marshmallow root.

COUGHS AND SORE THROATS

Marshmallow and Liquorice Cough Syrup

If using dried marshmallow root:
4 tbsp dried marshmallow root, chopped roughly
2 dried liquorice roots, broken up into small pieces
3 heads/bunches fresh elderberries
1 tsp cloves
peel of 1 mandarin
1 tsp aniseed seeds
1 sprig fresh eucalyptus leaves (about 8)
500 ml water
100 ml honey
juice of 1 lime
5 tbsp glycerine

If using fresh marshmallow root:
8 tbsp fresh marshmallow root, chopped roughly
4 dried liquorice roots, broken up into small pieces
other ingredients as above

1 Put the marshmallow, liquorice, elderberries, cloves, mandarin peel, aniseed and eucalyptus leaves into a pan with the water. Simmer until the liquid is reduced by one-fifth. Remove the liquorice and eucalyptus leaves and discard.

2 Blend the mixture in a liquidizer until smooth. Pour back into the pan and add the honey, lime juice and glycerine, then stir and simmer for 2 minutes.

3 Pour into sterilized, clear 250 ml bottles.

USE Take 2 tbsp, 3 times a day.
STORAGE Keep refrigerated. Use within 2 weeks.

Small red hawthorn berries (*Crataegus laevigata*), prolific in autumn hedgerows, have been shown in clinical studies to lower blood pressure, improve coronary blood flow and reduce the absorption of cholesterol in the body. Combined with artichoke (*Cynara scolymus*), which also contains cholesterol-lowering substances, this chewy fruit leather can help boost heart health, especially in those with borderline high levels of cholesterol. This makes a big batch – take a few pieces with you to munch on during the day.

CHOLESTEROL REDUCER
Hawthorn and Artichoke Fruit Leather

4 artichokes
1 litre water
475 g fresh hawthorn berries
225 g sugar
1 cinnamon stick
juice of 1 lime

1 Chop the artichokes, place in a saucepan, cover with the water and boil for 10 minutes, or until cooked. Remove from the heat, then leave to steep for 20 minutes. Strain into a bowl.

2 Heat the oven to 100°C.

3 Place the artichoke infusion, hawthorn berries, sugar and cinnamon stick in a pan, and bring to the boil. Simmer gently for 15–20 minutes, or until the mixture is soft. Take out the cinnamon stick and blend in a liquidizer with the lime juice, then pour into greased, lined baking trays to a thickness of about 1 cm.

4 Dry in the heated oven for 2–3 hours. (Check after 2 hours; you want it to be chewy, but not too tough.) Leave to cool, then slice into bite-sized pieces.

USE Chew on a piece of fruit leather whenever you like.
NB If high blood cholesterol is suspected, you must see a doctor. This recipe may be used in addition to, not as a substitute for, proper medical treatment.
STORAGE Keep in greaseproof paper in an airtight container in the refrigerator for up to 1 month.

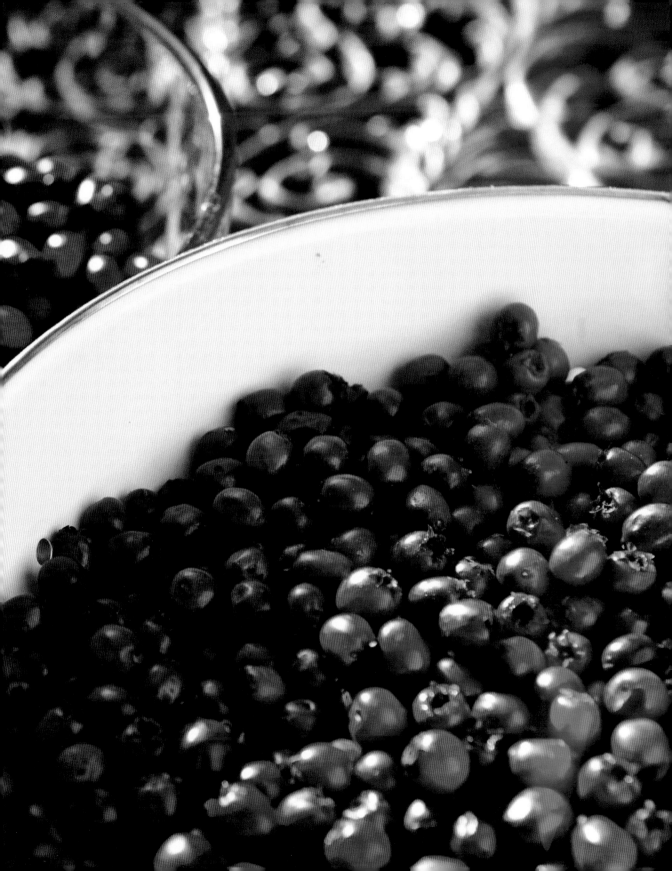

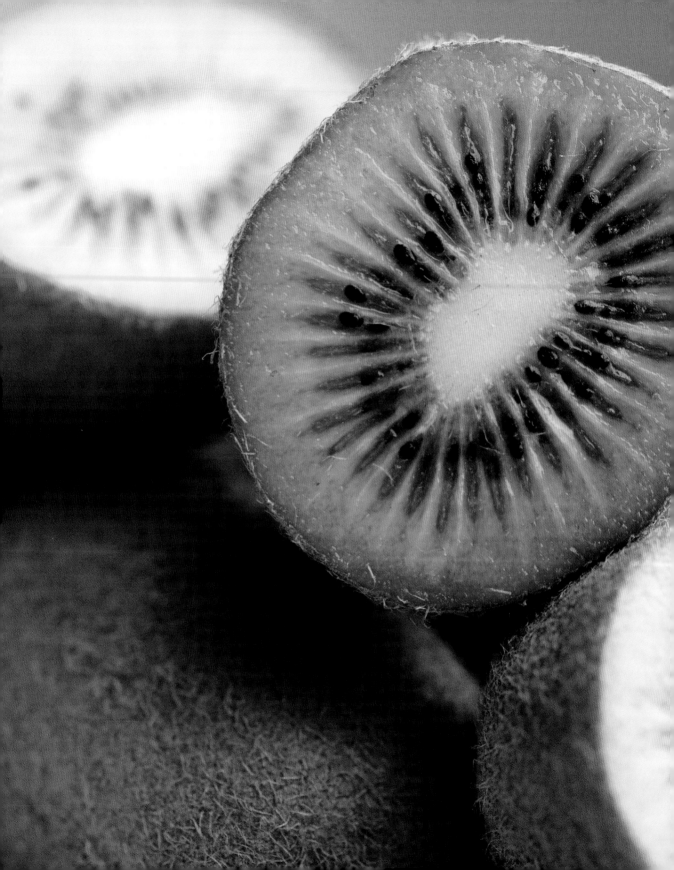

Kiwi fruit are high in vitamin C, which protects the liver, and feverfew (*Tanacetum parthenium*) is a gentle analgesic for headaches, so this smoothie is ideal for lifting morale the morning after the night before. Honey and kiwi fruit also contain fructose, a natural sugar shown to help alleviate hangovers.

HANGOVER

Kiwi Morning-after Smoothie

500 ml freshly boiled water
3 tbsp feverfew flowers
3 kiwi fruit, peeled
3 tbsp honey
½ tsp salt

1 Pour the water over the feverfew flowers and leave to steep for up to 8 minutes.

2 Place the infusion in a blender with the remaining ingredients and blitz until smooth. Add more honey to your taste – feverfew flowers can be bitter. Serve at once.

STORAGE Can be stored in the refrigerator for up to 24 hours.

Lemon balm can be effective at reducing the duration and frequency of cold sores. This balm is easy to carry round in a handbag or pocket and makes a good lip nourisher too. Use whenever you feel the need.

COLD SORES
Lemon Balm Lip Salve

21 tbsp (approx. 50 g) fresh lemon balm leaves
3 tbsp wheatgerm oil
115 ml olive oil
1 tbsp honey
1 tbsp beeswax
5 drops tea tree oil

1 Strip the lemon balm leaves and chop finely. In a pan over a slow heat, stir and crush one third of the lemon balm leaves with the wheatgerm and olive oil for 10 minutes, or until it starts to bubble. Take off the heat.

2 Strain the oil through a muslin-lined sieve or colander into a bowl, squeezing the leaves to get out all remaining juice. Throw away the squeezed leaves.

3 Repeat this process twice more with the remaining 2 batches of lemon balm leaves, using the same oil.

4 Place the oil in the pan on a gentle heat and add the honey and beeswax. Stir until melted, then take off the heat and stir in the tea tree oil.

5 Pour the salve into small sterilized jars, where it will set solid within 10 minutes.

USE Apply to cold sores whenever needed.
STORAGE Keeps for up to 1 year.

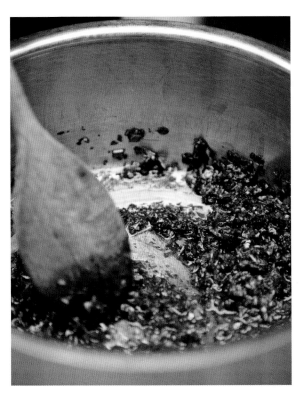

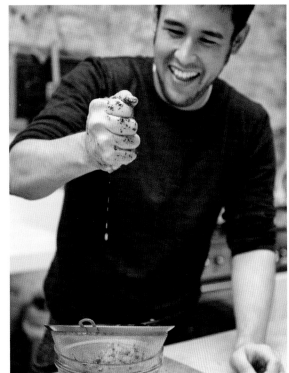

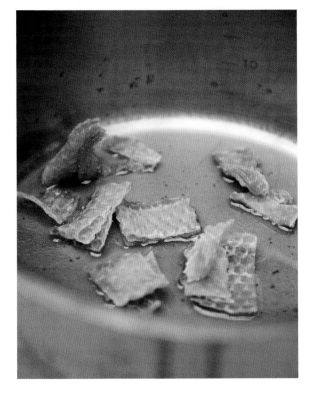

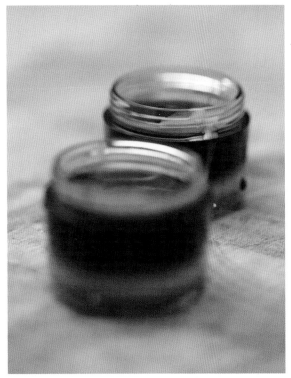

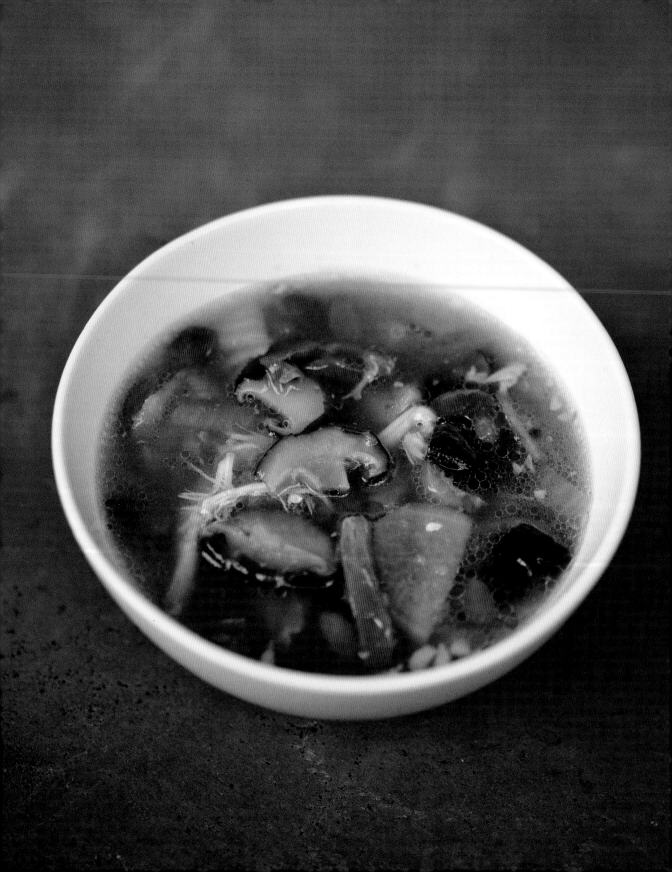

In China, soups rather than teas are the traditional way of administering health-giving herbs. This one is packed with nutrients that help to boost immunity and generally ease the symptoms of colds and flu. Eat this soup as soon as you feel a cold coming on.

IMMUNE SYSTEM BOOSTER
Goji Berry and Shiitake Soup

2 tbsp dried echinacea root
200 ml water, freshly boiled
5 tbsp goji berries, fresh or dried
2 litres chicken stock (homemade or from stock cubes)
3 chicken thighs or drumsticks (preferably organic)
2 large onions, peeled and sliced
12 shiitake mushrooms, thinly sliced
10 cm root ginger, peeled and shredded
2 fresh medium-sized chillies, finely sliced
8 garlic cloves, chopped
extra sliced ginger and chillis, to serve

1 Combine the dried echinacea root with the water in a bowl to make a simple infusion. In another bowl, pour just enough cold water over the goji berries to cover, and leave to rehydrate. Set the echinacea and goji berries aside and leave to stand.

2 Place the stock and chicken pieces in a large pan or slow cooker. Add the sliced onions, mushrooms, ginger and chillies and place around the chicken in the pan. On a very low heat, simmer gently for 1½–2 hours, or until the chicken is tender and falls apart. Take off the heat.

3 Five minutes before serving, add the goji berries and chopped garlic. Finally, strain the echinacea infusion and add this to the soup, reheating if necessary.

4 Serve by ladling into bowls and garnishing with sliced ginger and chilli for an extra kick.

USE Makes enough for 4. Can be eaten with noodles, if wished.

Honey is the magic ingredient in this soothing linctus,
but the cherries and lemon add a zingy punch of vitamin C.

COUGHS

Cherry Cough Syrup

500 g (approx.) cherries (leave the stones in)
1 lemon, sliced
250 ml honey

Put all ingredients in a pan with enough water to cover and simmer gently for about 30 minutes, or until the cherries are soft. Remove from the heat and strain out the solids, then allow to cool. Pour into a sterilized bottle.

USE Take 2 tbsp, as required, to soothe coughing.
STORAGE Keeps for several days in the refrigerator.

Mouth ulcers often arrive in clusters, making eating, drinking and even talking uncomfortable. Myrrh contains a painkilling resin that forms a film over the ulcers, while the peppermint and cloves are antiseptic and cooling. Used regularly for a couple of days, this mouthwash will improve symptoms and reduce discomfort.

MOUTH ULCERS
Myrrh Mouthwash

20 drops peppermint oil
5 drops clove oil
60 ml witch hazel
1 tsp tincture of myrrh (from chemists)
120 ml glycerine
250 ml cooled boiled or distilled water

Place all the ingredients in a bowl and stir well. Filter into a large sterilized bottle.

USE Dilute with warm water (1 part in 4) and use every hour as a mouthwash or gargle to relieve pain until the soreness has gone. Do not swallow in large amounts.
STORAGE Keeps for 1 month.

This is a good spring soup: the nettles (*Urtica dioica*) are packed with nourishing vitamins, minerals and chlorophyll, and help to build up natural immunity and protect from infections after a long winter.

RESTORATIVE

Nettle Soup

25 g butter
1 medium onion, finely chopped
2 garlic cloves, crushed
400 g potatoes, peeled and chopped
450 g freshly picked nettle tops (wear gloves to collect)
1 litre vegetable stock
150 ml double cream
freshly grated nutmeg
salt and freshly ground black pepper

1 In a large pan, melt the butter and gently cook the onion and garlic for 10 minutes. Add the potatoes and nettles and fry for 2 minutes. Add the stock and cover, then bring to the boil and simmer for 15 minutes. Leave to cool.

2 Purée the ingredients with a handheld bender, then stir in the cream and season with a little nutmeg, salt and pepper. Reheat and serve at once.

USE Makes enough for 6.

VARIATION
Nettle Pesto

This is another simple, tasty way to get the benefits of *Urtica dioica*. The young spring tips are the most tender and tastiest. Just cook a big handful of the young nettle tips (about 150 g) in boiling water for about 2 minutes. Drain, then drop into a blender along with some freshly grated Parmesan, 2 chopped garlic cloves, a handful of pine nuts and about 80 ml olive oil. Whiz until smooth, then spoon over freshly cooked pasta and mix in well.

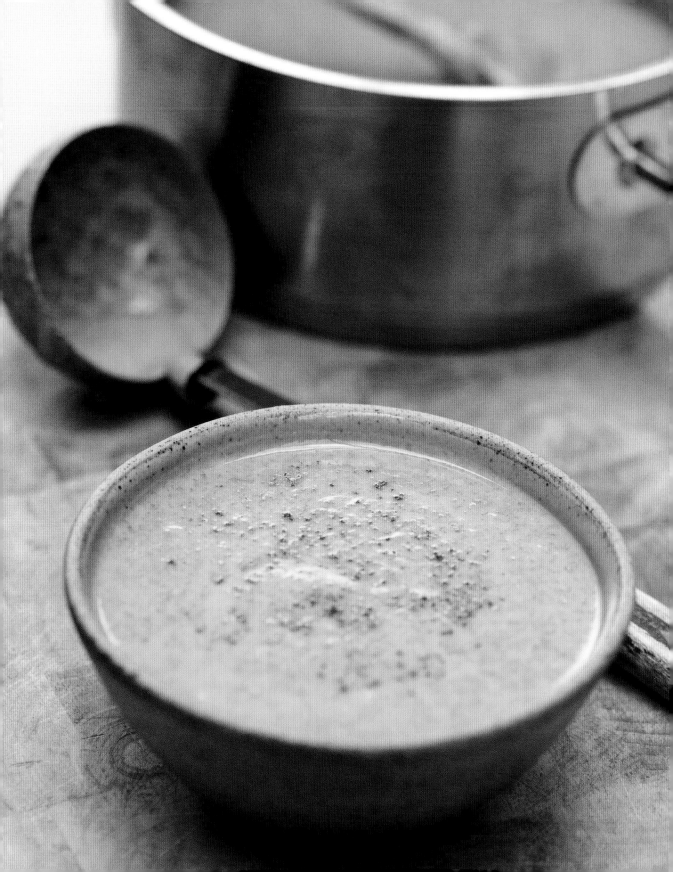

Echinacea has a beneficial effect on the immune system, as well as a numbing effect on the throat. Add the antiseptic properties of the cloves and sage and the cooling effect of the peppermint, and you'll get instant relief every time you use this spray.

SORE THROAT

Echinacea Throat Spray

3 cloves
5 peppermint leaves, finely chopped
5 sage leaves, finely chopped
30 ml *Echinacea purpurea* tincture
(from health food shops)

1 Place the cloves, peppermint and sage leaves in a small glass bowl, then add the echinacea tincture. Cover and leave to stand for 2 weeks in a cool, dark place. Gradually the colour will change.

2 Strain the liquid through a loose-weaved muslin placed in a strainer, squeezing all the liquid from the herbs by hand. Filter the liquid into a sterilized spray bottle.

USE Spray as often as needed.
STORAGE Keeps in the refrigerator for up to 1 year.

Pungent sage leaves (*Salvia officinalis*) contain antiseptic, anti-inflammatory and decongestant properties – in fact, so all-round helpful is this herb that it takes its name from the Latin verb 'to save'. Combined with the antibacterial and healing properties of honey, this makes a great throat soother.

SORE THROAT

Sage Honey

1 large bunch fresh sage leaves
enough runny honey (buy sage honey if you can),
   to cover the leaves

1 Wash and dry the sage leaves and place in a small pan with enough honey to cover. Simmer gently for 1 hour. Allow to cool to a temperature you can handle. (Be careful; sugar solutions and honey can become very hot and cause scalding.)

2 Strain the honey into a sterilized jar containing a sprig of sage, if desired.

USE Take 1 tsp whenever needed to soothe a sore throat. You can also use to sweeten and medicate hot lemon drinks for colds and flu; take 3–4 times a day when needed.
STORAGE Keeps for about 6 months.

MIND

Dried ginkgo leaves are now being widely used to help improve concentration, short-term memory and reaction time in the middle-aged to elderly. There has been an enormous amount of research into this herb recently, and many of its properties are now being demonstrated in clinical studies. It is not suitable for severe memory loss in Alzheimer's disease but can help with 'normal' forgetfulness.

MEMORY ENHANCER
Ginkgo Tea

2 tsp dried/5 fresh ginkgo leaves per cup
1 drinking cup freshly boiled water

Add the ginkgo leaves to the cup of freshly boiled water and steep for 10 minutes. Strain, and drink immediately.

USE Drink this tea once or twice a day.

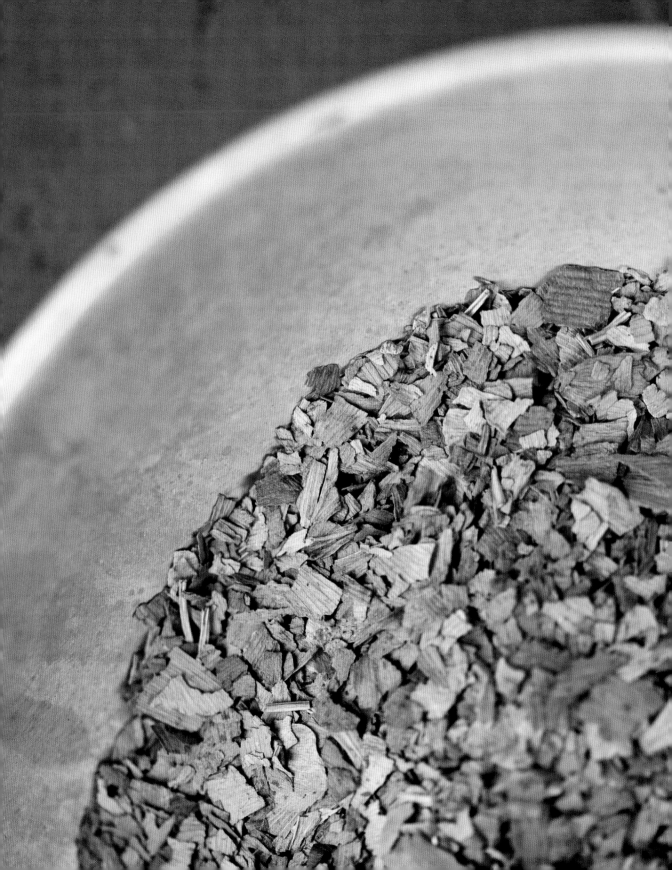

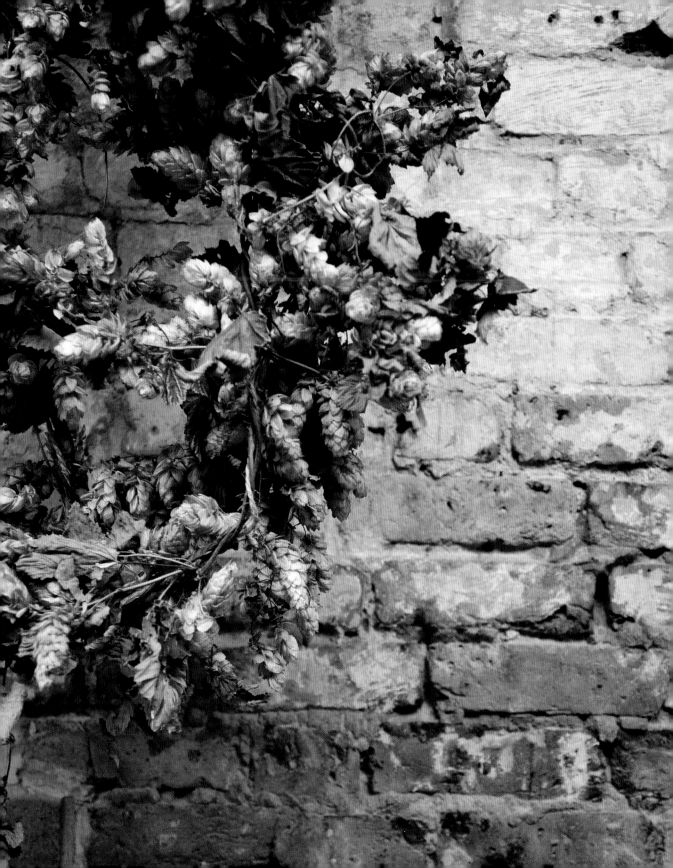

Sleeplessness – difficulty falling asleep or staying asleep – affects 30 per cent of us at some time in our lives. Hops flowers (*Humulus lupulus*) are renowned as a sleep promoter. They contain bitter acids and volatile oils that work together to soothe the nerves and relax, giving a better night's sleep without the after-effects of prescription sleeping medications. Dry your own hops freshly if possible (see step 1 below), to retain more of the volatile oils than are normally present in bought preparations.

INSOMNIA

Hops Pillow for Insomnia

For a pillow about 32 x 23 cm:
4 handfuls dried hops flowers
4 handfuls dried lavender flowers

1 To dry the hops and lavender yourself, tie them in bunches and hang upside down in a well-ventilated space out of direct sunlight for 2 weeks. Alternatively, place in a low oven (about 100ºC) for 30 minutes or so until dry and crispy. Strip the flowers off the larger or harder stalks.

2 Put equal handfuls of dried hops and lavender flowers into a cotton pillowcase, and seal the end.

USE Place the pillow under or beside your head to induce sleep.

VARIATION
Chamomile and Hops Bath

1 To make a small muslin bag, place together two small squares of muslin and sew together three sides. Put 1 handful (approx. 20 g) chamomile flowers and 1 handful (approx. 20 g) hops into the bag, then sew up the opening. Alternatively, use a clean pop sock or cut the foot off a pair of tights, and tie the top.

2 Put the bag into the bath while the water is running, swishing it around the bath and squeezing occasionally. The hot bath water allows the relaxing oils in these herbs to vaporize and be inhaled.

3 Relax in the bath for at least 15–20 minutes.

Feverfew (*Tanacetum parthenium*) was mentioned in *The British Herbal* in 1772, where Sir John Hill extolled its virtues for use with 'raging' headaches. Clinical studies have since shown that the fresh leaves are highly effective at preventing migraine, if taken regularly. You can grow the plant in your garden.

As the leaves taste bitter and unpleasant, it's best to add them to other food to disguise the flavour. Feverfew is also recommended for arthritic pains.

MIGRAINE PREVENTION
Feverfew Sandwiches

2 fresh feverfew leaves
sandwich, containing filling of your choice

To aid digestion, add two fresh leaves (1 g)
to a lunchtime sandwich.

Here is a simple, soothing drink to calm anxiety and promote sleep at the end of a stressful day. If you don't have valerian or lemon balm, don't worry – you will still enjoy it.

ANXIETY
Valerian Hot Chocolate

Makes 3 cups
3 tbsp fresh valerian root
3 tbsp fresh lemon balm leaves
3 tsp fresh lavender flowers
6 leaves and 3 heads from fresh passion flowers
peel of 1½ oranges
900 ml full-fat milk
50 g dark chocolate (minimum 50% cocoa solids)
dash of vanilla extract

1 Chop the top and bottom from the fresh valerian root. Add the valerian, lemon balm, lavender, passion flowers, orange peel, and milk to a pan and gently heat for 5–10 minutes. Strain.

2 Pour the infused milk back into the pan, then add the dark chocolate and vanilla extract and stir until melted. Drink at once.

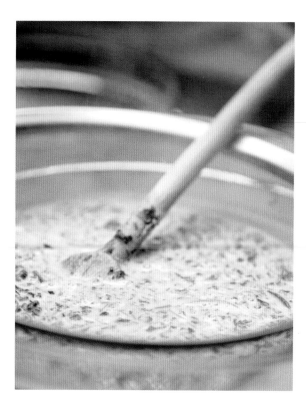
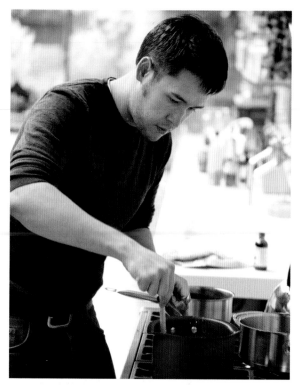
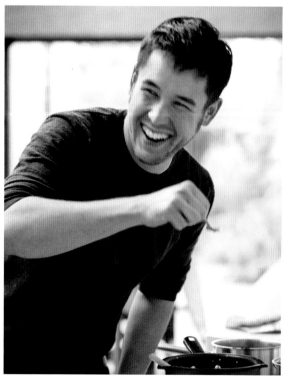
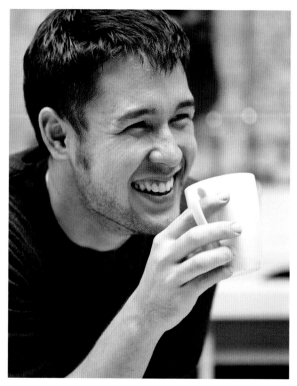

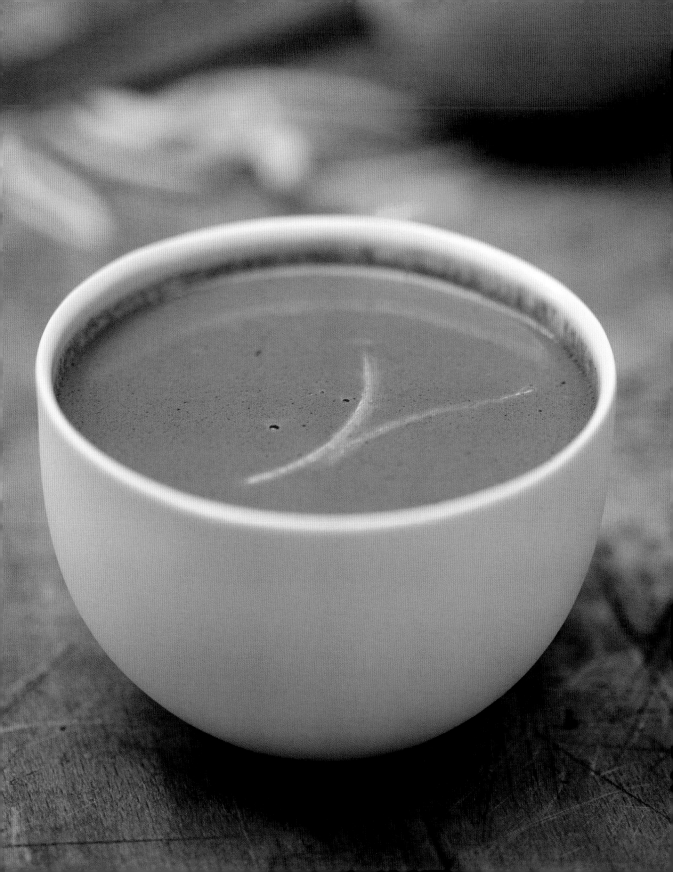

Rosemary is called the 'herb of remembrance' and has traditionally been used to improve memory and help with dementia. For this memory-boosting tonic it's best to use southern French or Californian wine (for the high alcohol content and warmth of the sun).

MEMORY BOOSTER
Rosemary Wine

1 bottle good-quality (preferably organic) wine
5 sprigs fresh rosemary

Bruise the rosemary and place in the bottle of wine. Recork and shake every day for 2 weeks.

USE Drink one small wine glass daily after dinner.

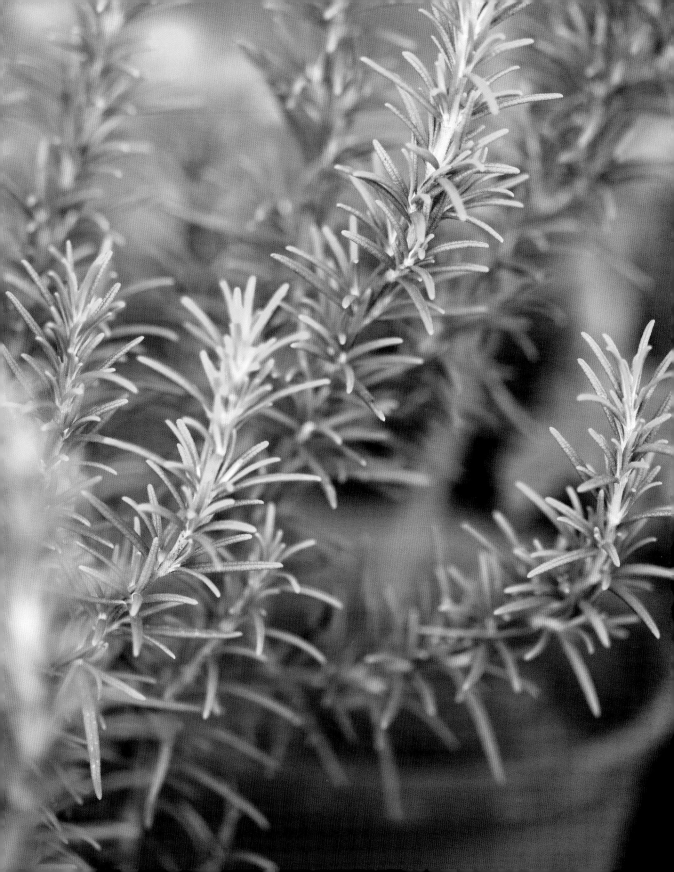

FACE AND BODY

An easy-to-make hair tonic that can be used as a final rinse after shampooing, or as a hair strengthener to stimulate growth. Either way, you'll be left with smooth, soft hair.

HAIR STRENGTHENER
Nettle Hair Tonic

1 large bunch nettle leaves, fresh or dried
500 ml water
500 ml white wine vinegar
1 tbsp aromatic herbs
   (eg rosemary, lavender) or 10 drops essential oil

Simmer the nettles in the water and vinegar for 2 hours, then stir in the aromatic herbs or essential oil and allow the mixture to cool. Strain through a sieve lined with fine-weaved muslin. Filter into bottles.

USE Apply to the scalp every other night as a hair-strenthening tonic, or use as a leave-in, final hair rinse after shampooing.
STORAGE Keeps for at least 1 month.

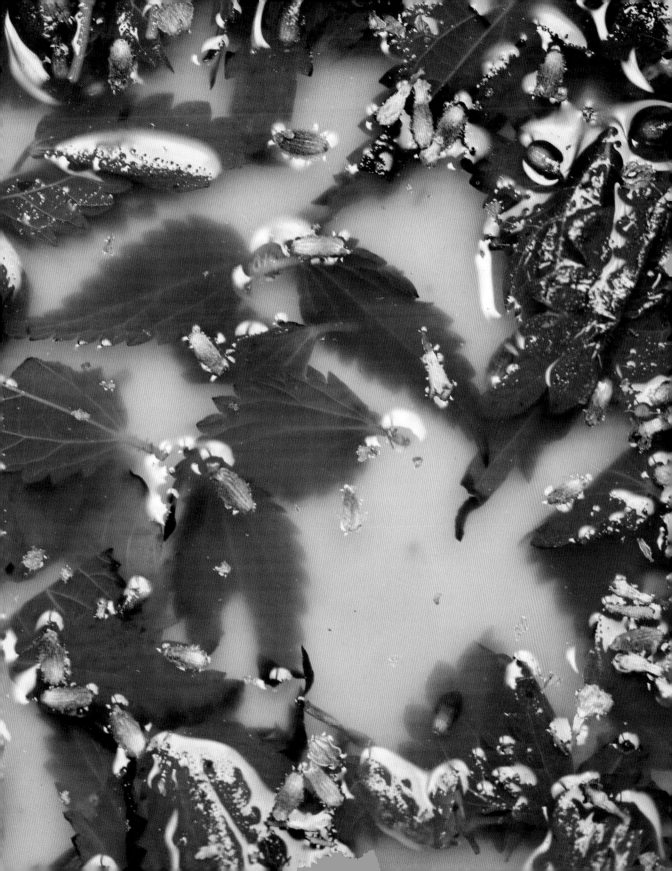

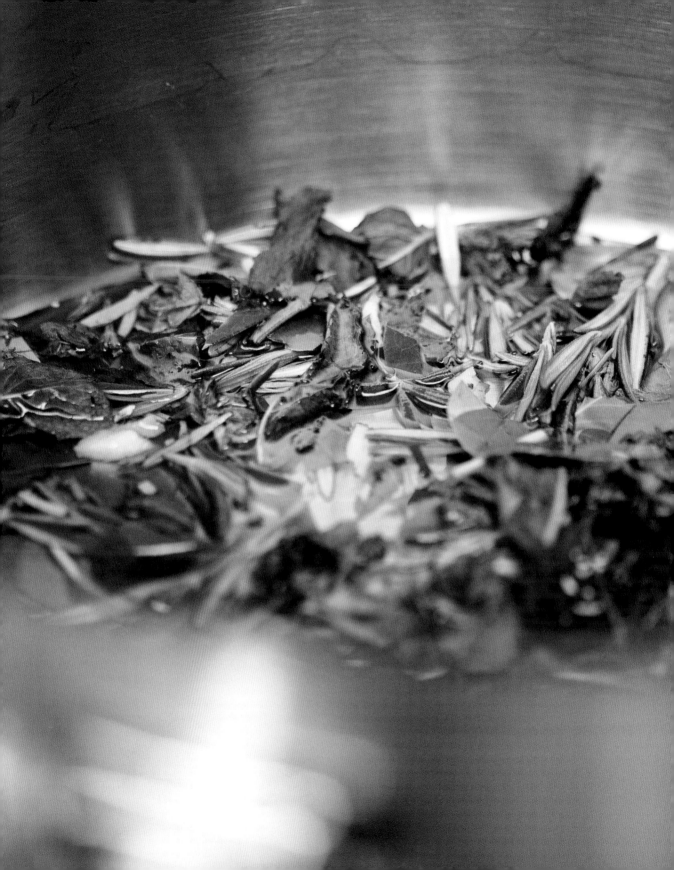

Combine the words 'cosmetic' and 'pharmaceutical' and you get 'cosmeceutical', the name for cosmetics that are supposed to have a biological effect on the body. To the West, cosmeceuticals are a new and trendy concept, but in most other medical traditions, medicine and cosmetics are one and the same – a patient is as likely to visit a shaman for limp, lacklustre hair as for indigestion. After all, a healthy person also looks good. This scrub might just seem cosmetic, but it stimulates the circulatory system, making you look good from the inside out.

BODY SCRUB
Herbal Scrub

50 g fresh mint leaves, finely chopped
50 g fresh eucalyptus leaves, finely chopped
50 g fresh rosemary leaves, finely chopped
1 tbsp freshly ground black pepper
peel of 2 lemons
300 ml olive oil
400 g sea salt (fine-grained)
4 tsp vitamin C powder
extra eucalyptus leaves and slices of lemon peel, to decorate

1 Place the chopped herbs, black pepper and lemon peel in a pan, then add the olive oil. Place on a medium heat and stir, then leave for 2 minutes. Place the paste in a piece of muslin over a sieve and squeeze out all the oil into a bowl below.

2 Mix the sea salt and vitamin C powder in a bowl. Add most of the oil (reserving a little to seal the jar) and stir well. Place the mixture in a sterilized Kilner jar and press down well. Decorate the top with a few eucalyptus leaves and slices of lemon rind. Pour a layer of the remaining oil on top of the salt scrub to keep it airtight.

USE Apply to wet skin in the bath or shower, when needed. Scrub, then rinse off well with warm water.
STORAGE Keeps for 6 months, or 1 year in the refrigerator.

This oil is soothing in baths or for massage, and you can also add it to a bowl of hot water for use as an inhalation.

BATH AND MASSAGE OIL
Pine and Eucalyptus Oil

¼–½ tsp pine or cedar resin
  (for stockists see Resources, page 219)
20 fresh eucalyptus leaves
2 tsp cloves
2 cinnamon sticks
200 ml almond oil

Place all the ingredients in a pan and gently heat for 20 minutes to macerate. Strain through a sieve lined with muslin. Pour into a sterilized bottle with a stopper.

STORAGE Keeps for up to 6 months in a dark, cool place.

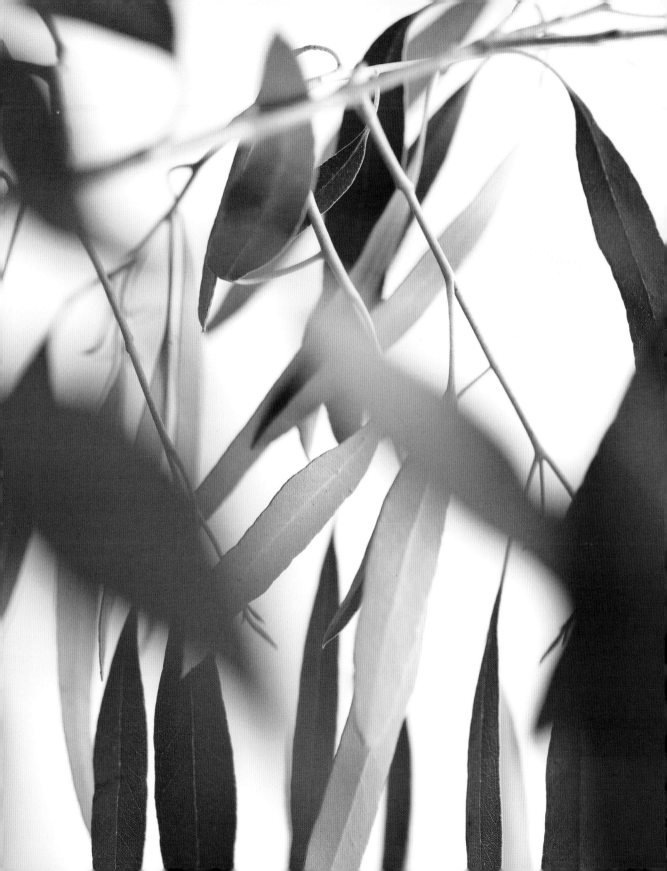

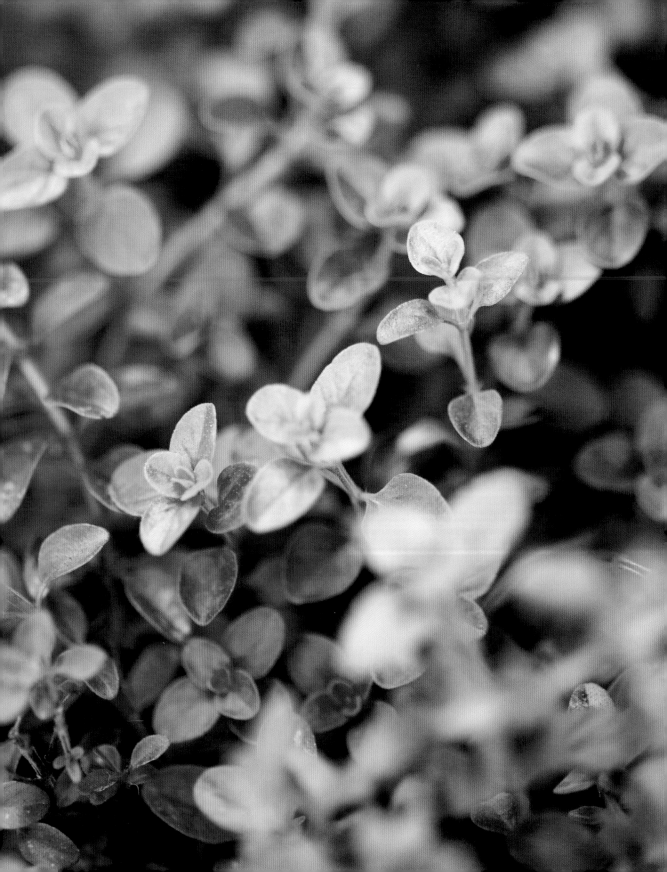

In the Middle Ages, people thought that bad smells caused certain diseases, and sweet scents had the power to cure them. The logic may be flawed, but there is some truth in the concept – bad smells usually come from dangerous bacteria, clean-smelling substances are often antibacterial, and we're evolutionarily hard-wired to respond to both. This natural, aluminium-free deodorant contains fragrant pine, which will help blitz odour-causing bacteria.

DEODORANT
Pine Spray

½ tsp pine resin (for stockists see Resources, page 219)
250 ml vodka (or just enough to cover the ingredients)
rind of 2 lemons, finely chopped
rind of 2 oranges, finely chopped
10 fresh bay leaves, finely chopped
3 tbsp fresh pine needles, finely chopped
3 tbsp fresh thyme leaves
2 tbsp glycerine
100 ml orange blossom water

1 Crush the pine resin in a pestle and mortar until you have a very fine powder. Pour over 1 tbsp of vodka and stir to dissolve. The mixture should form a thin paste. Add the chopped lemon and orange rind to the mortar and stir with a spoon to remove the last traces of sticky resin from the sides.

2 Place the resin mixture along with the bay leaves, pine needles and thyme in a Kilner jar. Add enough vodka to cover, then seal and leave in a dark place for 2 weeks to 1 month.

3 When ready, strain off the herbs through a muslin-lined sieve into a jug, and stir in the glycerine and orange blossom water. Pour into a 100 ml glass spray bottle.

USE Do a 24-hour test on a small patch of skin before using. Shake well and apply every morning to underarms, feet, etc.
STORAGE Keeps for up to 1 year in a cool, dry place.

A gel mask that harnesses the natural fruit acids in kiwi fruit, lime and papaya to exfoliate gently, leaving the skin smooth and rejuvenated. Makes enough for 1–2 face masks.

FACE MASK

Kiwi and Papaya Face Mask

1 kiwi fruit, peeled
juice of 1 lime
½ papaya
2 sachets vegetable gelatine

1 Mash the kiwi fruit through a sieve into a bowl. Add the lime juice to the kiwi mixture.

2 Scoop the seeds from the papaya, and mash the flesh on a chopping board using a fork (this makes it slightly easier to press through the sieve). Press the papaya through a sieve into a separate bowl and mix with the vegetable gelatine using a fork.

3 Put the bowl with the papaya mixture over a saucepan of boiling water and stir constantly until it forms a wallpaper-paste consistency. Take off immediately and continue to stir. Add the kiwi fruit juice slowly, bit by bit, stirring all the time. Leave to cool.

USE When cool or lukewarm, apply the gel to face, avoiding the eye area, and leave for 10 minutes to 1 hour. Wash off with warm water.

STORAGE Most effective when used as soon as possible. Keeps in the refrigerator for up to 48 hours.

VARIATION
Lemon Jelly Peeling Face Mask

This mask uses everyday ingredients from the kitchen. Soak ½ sliced cucumber in 125 ml lemon juice for 30 minutes in a heat-resistant bowl. Sprinkle 1 tbsp vegetable gelatine into the juice. Place the mixture in the microwave and heat on a low setting until the gelatine dissolves completely. Leave until cool enough to handle. Spread over the face, avoiding the eye area. Leave on for 20 minutes, then wash off with warm water.

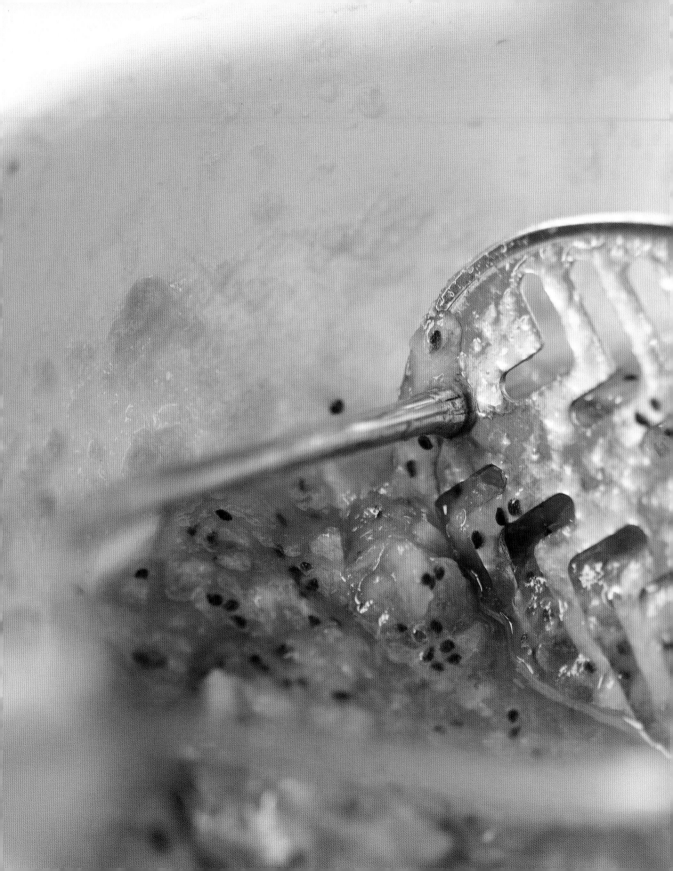

A sweet-smelling and nourishing hand cream
that's quick and easy to make.

HAND CARE
Rich Hand Oil

4 tsp avocado oil
2 tsp evening primrose oil
2 tsp vitamin E oil
5 drops sandalwood essential oil
5 drops lemon essential oil
5 drops geranium essential oil

Put all the ingredients into a bowl and mix
thoroughly. Place in a sterilized balm jar
and seal.

USE Massage a small amount into hands
and feet as needed.
STORAGE Keeps for up to 6 months in
a cool, dark place.

This is a flexible recipe, in which you can substitute other dried flowerheads and essential oils. You'll need a large biscuit cutter to shape the bomb – ideally 3–4 cm wide and about 3 cm deep. Children will love helping you make this.

BATH BOMB
Lavender Bath Bomb

5–6 fresh lavender sprigs
1 tbsp citric acid powder
3 tbsp bicarbonate of soda
10 drops lavender essential oil
1 tsp plant-based oil (vegetable or almond oil)

1 Heat the oven to 180ºC. Once it has reached that temperature, turn it off and place the lavender, hanging upside down, in the oven to dry for about 2 hours. When dry, remove the flowers from the stalks and set aside.

2 For the next stage you need to make sure that the bowl you are using, and your hands, are completely dry – otherwise the bomb will start fizzing. In a glass bowl, mix the citric acid and bicarbonate of soda together. Add a few drops of lavender oil and 1 tsp dried lavender flowers, along with the vegetable or almond oil. Mix everything together with a metal spoon.

3 Place the biscuit cutter on top of a sheet of baking paper. Put the mixture into the biscuit cutter and press down with the back of the spoon. The oil now needs to evaporate so the bomb can set as a dry, hard block – leave for a minimum of 30 minutes and preferably overnight.

STORAGE Store in tin foil to keep out moisture.

VARIATION
If you are making this with kids you can add ½ tsp of edible glitter into the mix to create an even more dramatic effect.

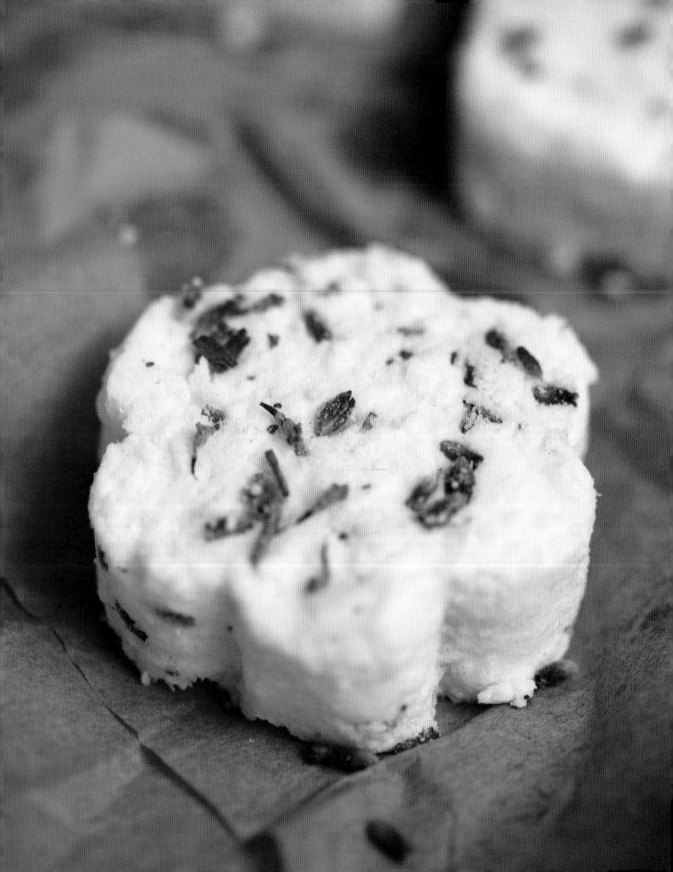

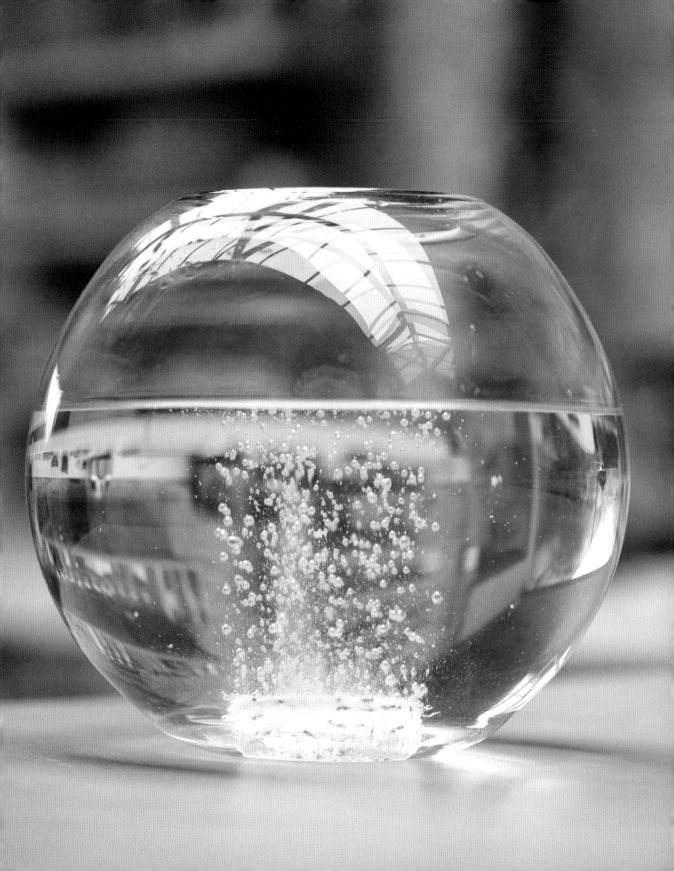

A gentle exfoliator for use once a week. The basil oil kills bacteria and the almonds, oats and vinegar slough off dead cells to leave skin feeling softer and looking clear and bright.

EXFOLIATOR
Rejuvenating Face Scrub

1 tsp ground almonds
1 tsp oat flakes
pinch of salt
½ tsp cider vinegar
2 drops basil essential oil

Mix all the ingredients in a small bowl. With dampened fingers roll the mixture over the face, then rinse off.

This is a very old recipe touted as a cure-all for internal and external use. It is certainly a good toner for the face or a hair rinse (if made with vinegar), and it makes a fragrant eau de cologne (if made with vodka).

FACE TONER/HAIR RINSE
The Queen of Hungary's Water

6 parts fresh lemon balm leaves
4 parts German chamomile (*Matricaria recutita*) flowers, fresh or dried
3 parts marigold (*Calendula officinalis*) flowers, fresh or dried
4 parts rosebuds or petals, fresh or dried
1 part rosemary leaves, fresh or dried
1 part lemon peel
1 part sage leaves
1 part fresh lovage root
apple or wine vinegar, or vodka, to cover
3 drops lavender or rose essential oil

1 Crush all the fresh leaves and flowers, slice the lemon peel and lovage root, and place together in a Kilner jar. Add enough vinegar or vodka to cover the plant matter, then seal the jar. Shake every day for 2 weeks.

2 Strain through a sieve lined with two layers of muslin. Add a couple of drops of lavender or rose essential oil, then filter into bottles.

USE Use as a facial toner, as a final hair rinse, or dab on as eau de cologne (with the vodka version).
STORAGE Keeps for up to 1 year in a dark, cool place.
NB Heat and light will destroy the fragrance.

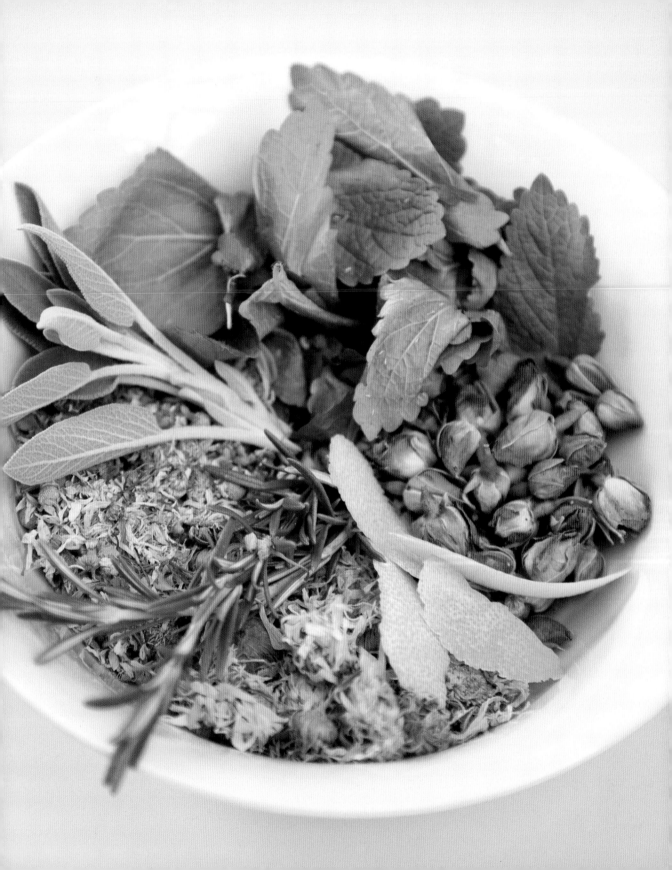

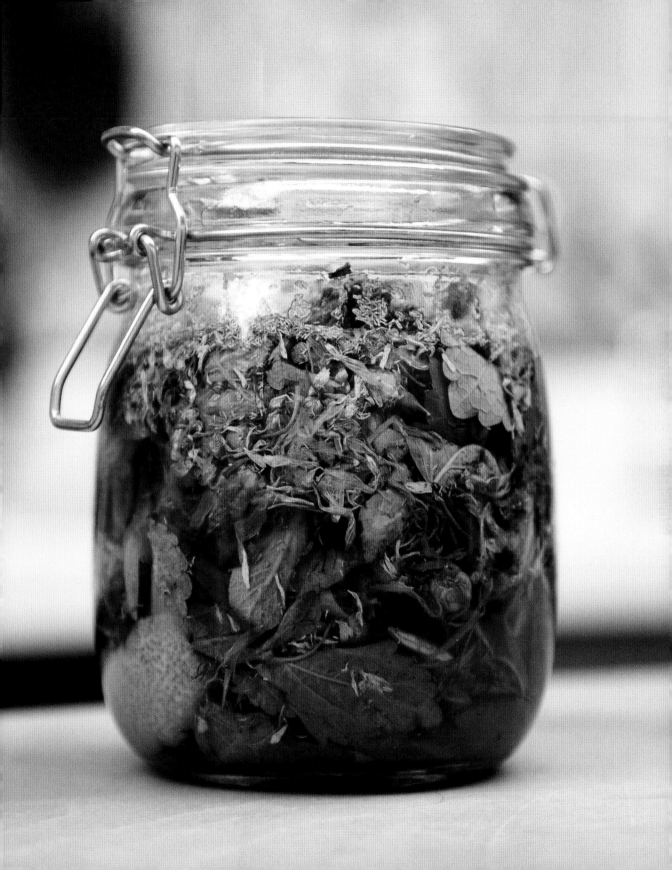

A cooling gel to soothe sore or swollen eyes.

FOR SORE EYES
Cucumber Eye Gel

1 small cucumber, chopped
1 aloe vera leaf
1 sachet vegetable gelatine
50 ml distilled extract of witch hazel BP
1 white tea teabag
3 drops peppermint essential oil

1 Roughly chop the cucumber. Peel and slice the aloe leaf to extract its gel. Put the cucumber and aloe gel into a blender and process until smooth. Strain the mix through a sieve to extract the juice. Measure out 100 ml of the strained juice and set aside.

2 Add the witch hazel to a pan, whisk in the gelatine and add the teabag. Gently heat the mixture until it just starts to thicken. As the mixture cools, take out the teabag, then whisk in the cucumber and aloe juice mixture and the peppermint oil.

3 Bottle up the gel in a sterilized, airtight pump dispenser.

USE Apply to the eye area before bed, then wash off in the morning.
STORAGE Keeps in the refrigerator for up to 6 weeks.

A refreshing lotion to soothe tired, red eyes at the end of the day. Eyebright (*Euphrasia officinalis*) has a long history of use for eye conditions.

FOR TIRED OR RED EYES

Eyebright Eye Wash

1 tbsp dried eyebright
600 ml water

Place the eyebright in a small pan and add the water. Bring to the boil and simmer for 10 minutes. Strain carefully through muslin (the liquid should be clear). Leave to cool, then pour into a glass bottle or jar.

USE Use undiluted in an eyebath 3–4 times a day.
STORAGE Keeps for 1 week in the refrigerator.

VARIATION
Chamomile and Marigold Eye Lotion

This sweet-smelling eye lotion is packed with soothing anti-inflammatories, great for at the end of a heavy day in front of a computer screen.

1 Take 1 tsp each of chopped German chamomile and marigold (*Calendula officinalis*) flowers, rose petals and fennel seeds, and place in a glass bowl. Pour over 500 ml hot (not boiling) water and steep the herbs for 30 minutes.

2 Strain carefully through a double layer of muslin, then filter again, to give a very clear lotion. Pour into a sterilized glass bottle. Use in an eyebath (diluted with a little warm water) 3–4 times a day. Keeps for 1 week in the refrigerator.

Remedies: Face and Body

Want a simple, natural soap that doesn't irritate dry or sensitive skin? Glycerine attracts moisture into the skin, leaving it feeling softer and more nourished. This soap is good for delicate and mature skins, and also looks pretty studded with rosebuds and petals.

GLYCERINE SOAP
Gentle Soap

Makes about 15 small soaps
500 ml flower water, such as orange or rose
500 ml glycerine
½ bar unperfumed white soap, grated
50 drops rose geranium essential oil
1 handful rose petals, chopped, or rose buds (optional)

1 In a glass bowl over a saucepan of boiling water, place the flower water, glycerine and grated soap. Stir continuously until the soap dissolves, then take off the heat. Add the rose geranium essential oil, and mix well. Drop the rose petals or buds into the mixture, if using, and stir.

2 Pour into moulds (you can buy these online) or make a soap 'loaf' by pouring into a small square or rectangular straight-sided china dish, making sure the petals and buds are evenly distributed throughout. Leave to cool for at least 2 days. Cut the soap loaf into bars before use.

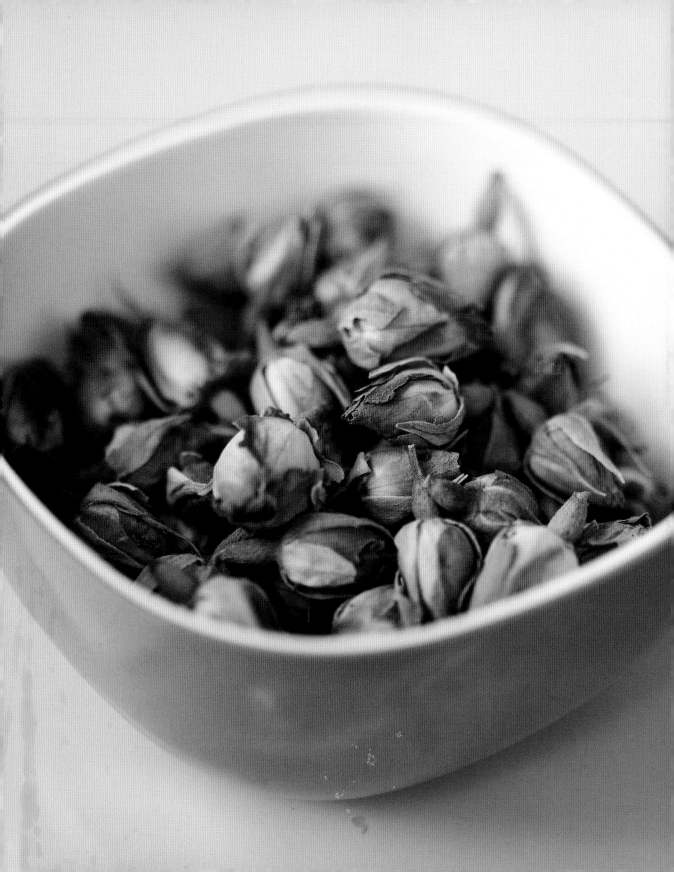

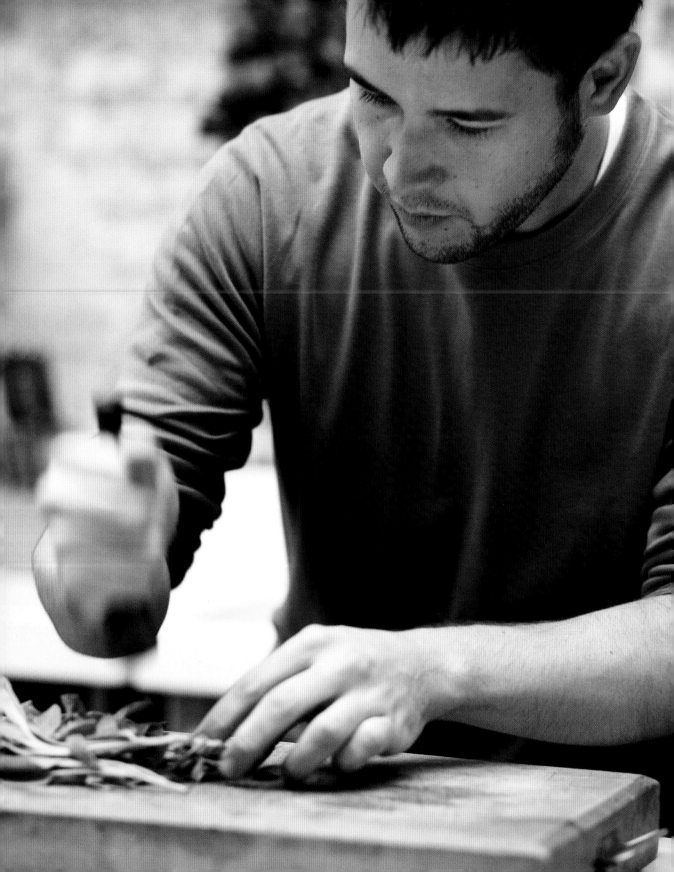

A good germ-killing toothpowder, which has antiseptic and astringent properties (from the sage), thus reducing and soothing swollen gums. Non-abrasive, it will remove plaque and freshen breath without damaging enamel, so can be used by all ages.

PLAQUE REMOVER AND GUM SOOTHER

Sage and Sea-salt Toothpowder

350 g sea salt
100 g fresh sage leaves

1 Pound the salt and sage leaves.

2 Bake the mixture on the lowest oven setting until it dries out thoroughly (do not allow to burn). This will take at least 20 minutes but you will need to check from time to time because it depends on the oven temperature and salt.

3 Grind to a fine powder in a coffee or salt grinder (this is easy once the mixture is dry), then put in a shallow, wide-mouthed sterilized jar with a lid to keep airtight.

USE Use as normal toothpaste, to brush teeth morning and night.
STORAGE Keeps very well if stored in an airtight container. Use until the aroma of sage has gone.

Lip balms are easy to make, and this one is nourishing and gently antiseptic. It will stop lips getting chapped and sore – or rescue them if they already are. Make sure you use scented, organically grown roses – unscented varieties may not have the necessary properties and it's best to avoid the chemicals used on many commercially grown roses.

CHAPPED LIPS
Beeswax Lip Balm

For the herb oil:
1 large handful (approx. 20 g) rose or marigold (*Calendula officinalis*)
   petals (scented and organically grown)
250 ml almond oil

For the lip balm:
250 ml rose or marigold oil, see above
2–3 tbsp beeswax
1 tsp runny honey
1 tsp vitamin E oil
1 tsp aloe vera gel – from the centre of fleshy leaves, optional

1 Soak the rose or marigold petals in the oil for at least 5 days, in full sunlight in summer or in a warm place in winter. Strain through a fine-mesh sieve lined with muslin while the liquid is slightly warm, squeezing the petals to extract the oil and scent.

2 Warm the oil in a glass bowl over a pan of hot water and add the beeswax while stirring continuously. When dissolved, add the honey, vitamin E oil and aloe vera gel (if using), stirring all the time. Pour into a small, sterilized balm jar with a wide neck, and cap tightly. The balm will harden as it cools.

USE Apply when needed to chapped or cracked lips.
STORAGE Keeps at least 6 months, preferably in a refrigerator.

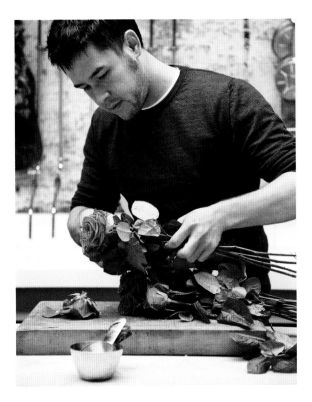
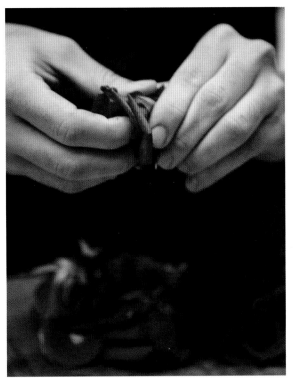
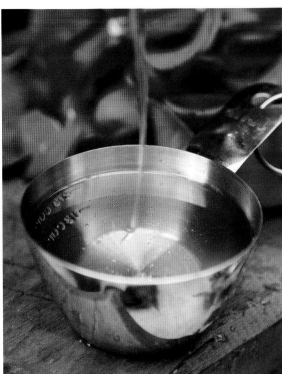
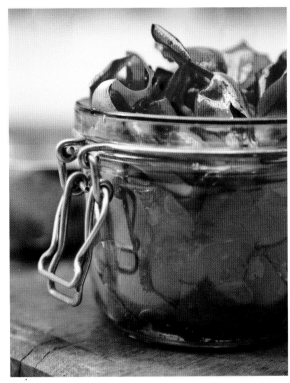

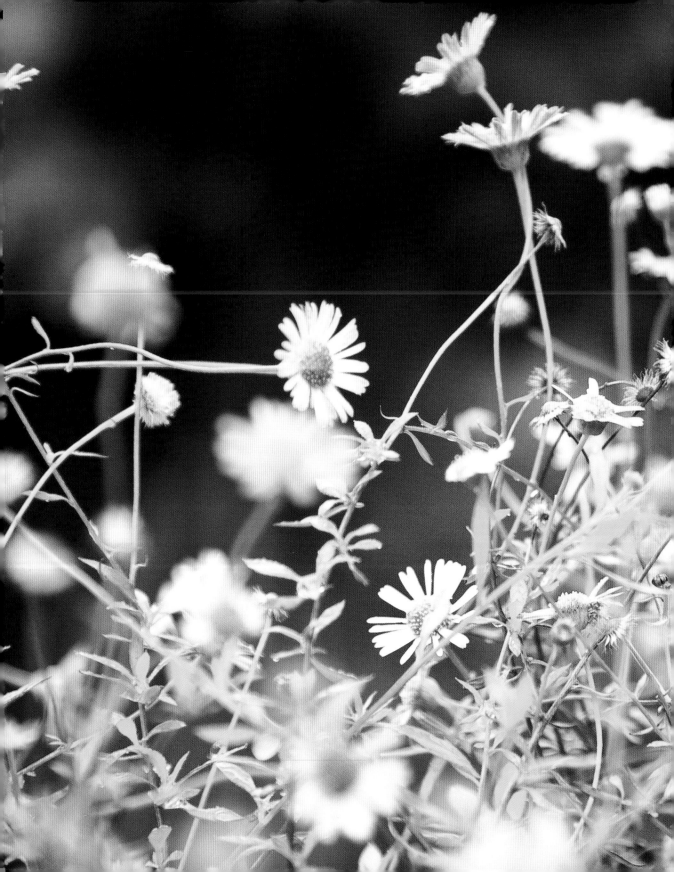

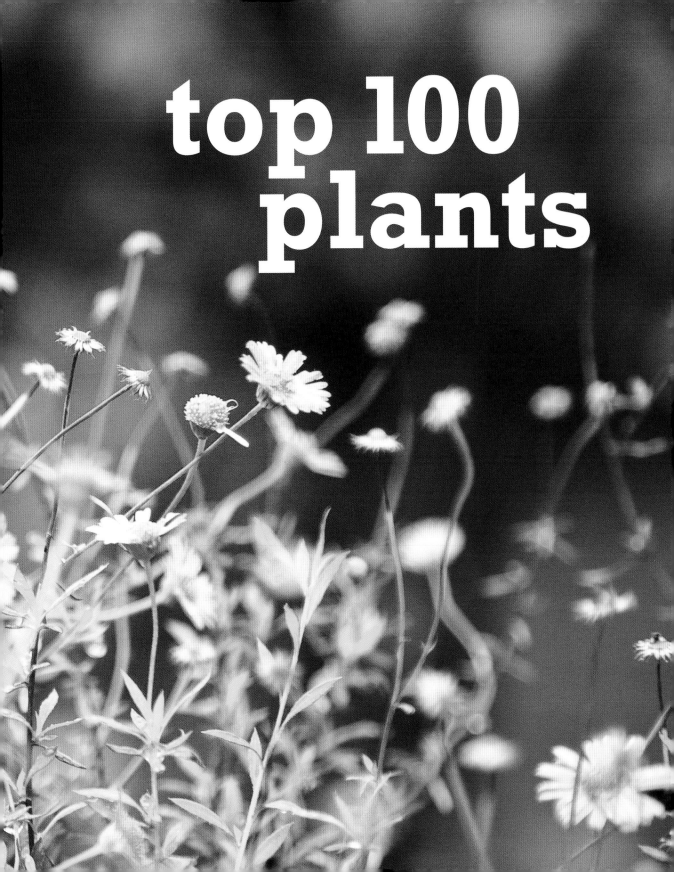

top 100
plants

The biggest challenge to those new to making herbal remedies is the sheer number of potential medicinal plants to choose from – with scientists' latest estimates clocking in at up to 50,000 species. With unpronounceable Latin names, and unfamiliar growing techniques at every turn, how do you know where to start?

The good news is that a huge number of the most useful species are also conveniently familiar, and are probably already growing in your window box or between the cracks of your patio or sitting in your spice rack. Mint, thyme, chillies, garlic and even dandelions and nettles might not seem like cutting-edge drugs, but trapped within the cells of these species are biologically active chemicals with proven medicinal properties – many of which are commonly found in over-the-counter drugs.

But perhaps the most exciting news for horticultural novices is that medicinal herbs are normally the easiest of plants to grow. In fact, many are actually invasive weeds in their country of origin – meaning that if you can grow a weedy nettle, you can grow a medicinal herb garden. You don't need a huge plot or hours of dedication, either: herbs can be grown in any spot with water, light and air, whether that's a sprawling country estate or a tiny window box. In fact, I've grown herbs like basil, mint and watercress in glasses of water on a kitchen window sill. Just pop a couple of cut stems into a glass, and treat exactly like you would a vase of flowers, and they will quickly produce roots and grow away happily for months on end.

To get you started, we have created an index of the Top 100 medicinal plants. And anyone can have a go at growing these or, in some, cases buying them from the greengrocer, supermarket or other supplier (see the Resources section on page 219). Once you have exhausted these, you might want to make a start on the other 49,900 other species.

FRUIT

Aniseed
Pimpinella anisum

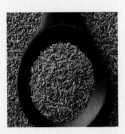

Aniseed is the fruit of a small annual plant grown widely in warmer parts of the world. Its liquorice-like smell and sweet flavour make it popular as a cooking spice and to flavour confectionery like aniseed balls and alcoholic drinks like raki. Aniseed helps loosen upper-respiratory congestion and is often used in cough medicines and lozenges (see Marshmallow and Liquorice Cough Syrup, page 103).

It has traditionally been used as a digestive aid, helping to soothe dyspepsia, colic, bloating and wind, and to control nausea and vomiting. It's also reputed to increase libido – it has mild oestrogenic properties and in some cultures is given to breastfeeding mothers to increase milk production. And it's a good, all-round odour-buster that masks unpleasant smells and is used to help freshen breath (see Thyme Sweet Breath Spray and Mouthwash, page 42). NB Do not use during pregnancy.

GROWS/WHERE TO FIND
→ health food shops

Bilberry
Vaccinium myrtillus

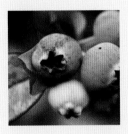

The blue–black fruits of the bilberry – or whortleberry, as it's sometimes called – is a summer delicacy that achieved mythic status after World War II, when British fighter pilots reported increased night vision after eating bilberry jam. Although that claim is unsubstantiated, trials have shown bilberry tincture to have very positive effects on eye health, especially on eye disorders caused by high blood pressure or diabetes. It can also help prevent cataracts and lessen glaucoma. The active ingredients are antioxidants and free-radical scavengers called anthocyanosides, which are also anti-inflammatory and anti-ageing. These have been shown to help significantly with vascular problems such as varicose veins and piles, as well as extremely painful periods (dysmenorrhoea) and water retention. The leaves can be made into a tea (see Using Plants, page 34), which is a popular remedy for diarrhoea and stomach cramps.

GROWS/WHERE TO FIND
→ best in acid soil – or it will yellow and do badly
→ doesn't like being moved
→ if potting, place in large pot
→ does better in exposed site
→ fruits best in full sun
→ buy from greengrocers during short late-summer season

Blackcurrant
Ribes nigrum

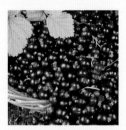

Blackcurrant oil is the richest plant source of gamma-linolenic acid (GLA). (The best source is borage oil.) It's used to treat long-lasting inflammatory skin conditions like eczema, as well as PMS, breast pain, mild hypertension and rheumatic disorders. Blackcurrant oil outperforms evening primrose oil for rheumatoid arthritis, though it needs to be taken over 6 months for best effect. As the oil comes from the seeds, it's probably easier to buy rather than make at home, as you'll need very large quantities of fruit. You can, however, make the leaves into tea (see Using Plants, page 34) for use as a mild diuretic, to lower blood pressure and alleviate inflammatory sore throats. The berries themselves are also antiviral, protecting against flu.

Blackcurrant Gargle: heat 2 tbsp blackcurrant leaves, chopped finely, in a pan with 250 ml water. Cover and simmer for 15 minutes. Strain, then cool. Use twice a day.

GROWS/WHERE TO FIND
→ easy to grow
→ full sun
→ add lots of organic matter to soil for high nitrogen levels during growing season
→ fruits on 1-year-old wood
→ prune old wood back in autumn
→ don't grow near pine trees, because these harbour damaging rust/fungus
→ net to prevent birds stripping
→ buy seed oil from health food shops

Black Mustard Seeds
Brassica nigra

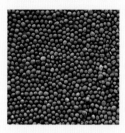

Mustard has a very hot flavour, and when applied on the body it also works by heating. It's a counter-irritant, causing reddening of the skin as blood rushes to the spot, and this increased blood flow can help reduce inflammation. Mustard plasters – a strong poultice of crushed mustard seeds and flour (see also Chilli Plasters, page 91) – were traditionally applied to the chest to bring relief from chesty colds, bronchial infections and rheumatic pains. The essential compounds are found in the seeds, which are produced in black pods borne by the striking yellow flowers in late summer. Add just a few drops of seed oil to a massage oil base and rub into stiff joints, aching muscles and cold extremities to improve circulation. Be cautious: mustard seed is extremely powerful and can cause skin iritation or burns. But in the right amount, you'll find it invigorating.

To make a reviving foot bath for sore feet, place 1–2 tbsp crushed seeds in a muslin bag or pop sock. Pour over 2 litres boiling water. Allow to cool a little, then soak feet for a few minutes. Rinse. (See also Hot Chilli and Mustard Foot Oil, page 70.)

GROWS/WHERE TO FIND
→ annual
→ easy to grow from seed
→ likes light soil and sunshine
→ harvest pods in late summer, tap to let the seeds out, then dry in a cool, well-ventilated space

Borage Seeds
Borago officinalis

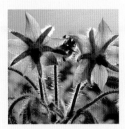

Borage grows like wildfire, its bright blue, star-shaped flowers spreading seed prolifically. It has been used for centuries in inflammatory and rheumatic conditions, to treat depression, as a diuretic and to promote sweating in fevers. Nowadays, the plant is cultivated mostly for its seeds, which are made into an oil known as starflower oil or borage seed oil. This oil is the richest plant source of gamma-linolenic acid (GLA) – greater than either evening primrose oil or blackcurrant oil. GLA is an omega-6 fatty acid used to treat dermatitis, arthritis, eczema, mastalgia, PMS, as well as the pain, tingling and numbness that can occur in diabetes.

Starflower oil can also reduce joint swelling, tenderness and pain in rheumatoid arthritis, and improve the condition and function of skin, especially in the elderly. It's easy to grow borage in the garden, but it's probably not worth it for the seeds – you need to take large regular doses of the oil (1–2 g of GLA, or 3–12 capsules a day, for at least 6 months). Buy it at your local chemist instead.

NB Don't take borage leaves internally because they contain compounds that can damage the liver. The flowers and seeds are safe, however.

GROWS/WHERE TO FIND
→ pharmacies

Caraway Seeds
Carum carvi

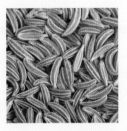

Caraway is not a common sight in this country despite being very easy to grow in gardens or pots. Umbrella-like clusters of tiny white blooms flower from June to August, and each flower stem contains two seeds. These are dried and used in herbal remedies to soothe stomach complaints in both children and adults. Caraway helps aid to digestion, ease griping pains, expel trapped wind and soothe bloating (see 'Four Winds' Tea, page 49). Mixed with peppermint oil, it reduces reflux so is also used for heartburn.

To dry caraway seeds: in late August or when seeds are ripe, cut plants at ground level, tie stalks in small bundles and hang upside down in a dry, well-ventilated space, with sheets of greaseproof paper below to catch the seeds.

GROWS/WHERE TO FIND
→ biennial
→ likes full sun
→ needs well-drained soil
→ sow seeds in September directly into ground or buy fledgling pot plants from nurseries
→ don't transplant because it hates root disturbance
→ self-seeds in autumn

Chaste Berry
Vitex agnus-castus

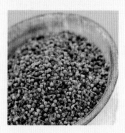

Although this aromatic plant is a native of the Mediterranean, it grows well in Britain, looking rather like a buddleia. Its prolific spikes of mauve flowers are followed in autumn by small, dark berries, which taste peppery and can be used fresh or dried in remedies. The berries are highly regarded as one of the best natural hormone-regulators for women. They contain a range of essential compounds that seem to raise levels of the hormone progesterone during the second half of the menstrual cycle – although the exact process is not yet understood. This has significant benefits for a wide range of disorders, relieving PMS and cyclical breast pain, helping with irregular bleeding, and diminishing hormone-related acne. In one study of infertile women, chaste berry extract taken for 3 months doubled the rate of pregnancies (from 10% to 21%). It's also suggested as a remedy to relieve menopausal symptoms.

Although chaste berries stimulate the female hormone system, they seem to have the opposite effect on men. Monks used to take the berries to reduce sexual desire and help them stay 'chaste', which is why they are also known as monk's pepper.

NB Don't use during pregnancy or while breastfeeding.

GROWS/WHERE TO FIND
→ shrub, grows to 5 m
→ does well in most soils
→ likes sun
→ purple flowers followed by dark fruits
→ you can buy standardized extracts (which have higher dosages than fresh berries) from health food shops

Cherry
Prunus avium

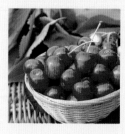

Sweet cherry trees grow wild in hedgerows and woods and are cultivated in gardens, and the fruit, stalks and even bark are used in a variety of sweet-tasting plant remedies. The fruit is packed with vitamins A, B and C, as well as the minerals calcium and magnesium, so it makes a good general immune-system booster in cold remedies and cough syrups. Cherry also has a reputation for lowering uric acid levels and has long been used in the treatment and prevention of gout and arthritis – though as yet there is no scientific evidence to support its use. Cherry stalks are anti-inflammatory and when taken as a tincture or tea can soothe dry, irritating coughs. The white inner bark can also be dried and made into a cough syrup though it will be tastier if you add some cherries for extra flavour. In large quantities, cherries are both diuretic and laxative – just don't eat too many at once.

Cherry Stalk and Apple Tea: put 30 g cherry stems, 3 apples (cored and sliced) and 1 litre water into a pan. Bring to the boil and simmer for 25 minutes, or until the apples are soft. Strain. Drink as a tea, 2–3 times a day, for dry and irritating coughs.

GROWS/WHERE TO FIND
→ likes full sun
→ grow beside a south- or west-facing wall
→ can be fan-trained
→ needs damp soil
→ self-sterile, so plant two varieties to ensure pollination
→ pick fruit when fully ripe (just before splitting)
→ harvest bark by pruning off small branches, stripping white inner bark and leaving to dry

Cranberry
Vaccinium macrocarpon

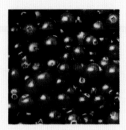

Cranberry is a sharp, sour fruit grown mostly in wet meadows in North America. Although best known as an accompaniment to Christmas lunch, it has a long history of treating cystitis and other urinary tract infections. It is thought to work by preventing bacteria from sticking to the lining of the urinary tract and increasing the acidity of urine. If you suffer recurrent bouts of cystitis, regularly eating Cranberry Fruit Leather (see page 99) or drinking homemade cranberry juice can help prevent further outbreaks (commercial juices are usually high in sugar). Cranberry is also used to help relieve the symptoms of acute attacks of cystitis, but you must check first with your GP to make sure it is cystitis and nothing more serious.

Cranberry and Apple Crush: put 115 g cranberries, 250 ml clear apple juice and 1 cup water in a pan and bring to the boil. Simmer until cranberries are soft. Strain well. Drink as often as required, adding a little sugar to taste.

GROWS/WHERE TO FIND
→ best in wet, acid soil
→ likes sun or light shade
→ can be grown in pots (don't allow to dry out)
→ best in open ground out of strong winds
→ buy from greengrocers or supermarkets

Elderberry
Sambucus nigra

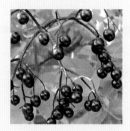

Elderflowers are often made into health-giving cordials and teas, but tiny black elderberries are less commonly used – perhaps because they have a very short season. However, the berries contain many of the same essential compounds as the flowers, and are traditionally used as an anti-inflammatory to soothe coughs, sore throats and bronchial infections and to make catarrh and sinus conditions looser and more productive. Elderberry has powerful antiviral properties that combat various flu strains and which have been shown to shorten the duration of flu attacks, so it is extremely useful for children and the elderly during the winter months. Take as a tincture or, for children, make into a syrup (see Using Plants, page 34). NB Don't eat unripe berries, which may cause vomiting and diarrhoea.

Elderberry Throat Gel: fill a small Kilner jar with ripe elderberries, then cover with diluted vegetable gelatine. Leave in a warm place for 2 weeks. Strain through muslin, squeezing well. Pour into a sterilized bottle. Adults: take 2 tsp, 3 times a day for coughs and sore throats.

GROWS/WHERE TO FIND
→ found wild in hedgerows and waste ground
→ easy to grow
→ vigorous – often considered a weed
→ fruit ripen best in full sun
→ harvest only ripe berries in September
→ strip berries from stems using a fork

Evening Primrose
Oenothera biennis

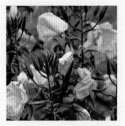

Evening primrose is a remarkable plant. During the day, it looks like any ordinary scrubland plant – in fact, it's classed as a weed in the United States, where it grows wild on wasteland and roadsides across the country. But in the evening, the yellow flowers open to welcome the moths that pollinate them overnight. Every part of the plant is edible: the nutty roots are boiled and eaten as vegetables; the leaves are eaten as greens; while the seeds were traditionally dried and chewed by Native Americans.

Today, the plant is cultivated mostly for its prolific seeds, cased in fluffy seed capsules, which are pressed to make evening primrose oil. Like borage, evening primrose oil is a rich source of gamma-linolenic acid (GLA), an essential fatty acid that can't be made in the body but which is essential for growth and bone health and to regulate metabolism.

Evening primrose is often recommended for the symptoms of premenstrual syndrome (sore breasts, irritability and bloating) and menopause. It has been shown to help with the itchiness, scaling and inflammation of eczema, to lower blood pressure slightly and to soothe ulcerative colitis.

For best effects, you'll need to take the oil internally for 6 months or more, but the plant is still worth growing for its unusual habits and edible roots and leaves.

GROWS/WHERE TO FIND
→ biennial
→ thrives on neglect
→ best in a low-nutrient soil
→ likes sun
→ buy oil from pharmacies

Fennel Seeds
Foeniculum vulgare

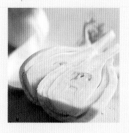

Fennel's beautiful feathery leaves and anise-flavoured bulbs are used in cooking, but it's the seeds that are prized in herbal remedies. Fennel relieves bloating, wind and tummy upsets of all kinds and it was a traditional ingredient in gripe water, used for centuries to soothe colic. It's also recommended for period pain and other menstrual disorders, perhaps because of its mild oestrogen-promoting qualities, and has been shown to increase breast milk flow in nursing mothers. If you're trying to lose weight, fennel might help: it has long been used as an appetite-suppressant. Make the seeds into a tea, tincture or oil (see Using Plants pages 34–5) and take every day.

Fennel Tea for Colic: place 1 tbsp fennel seeds in a pan with 400 ml water. Simmer for 10 minutes. Strain and cool. Give 1–2 tsp when needed, not more than twice per hour.

GROWS/WHERE TO FIND
→ likes a sunny spot
→ hates wet soil
→ can tolerate short drought
→ attracts wildlife, including slugs and snails
→ to dry seeds, gather flowerheads in late September/October, spread on greaseproof paper, and leave in warm, well-ventilated space, turning every few days. Shake or comb out

Figs
Ficus carica

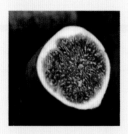

Syrup of figs has been used for hundreds of years as an effective and gentle laxative suitable for all ages. Figs work as a demulcent, soothing and protecting the gut, but are also nutritious and very high in soluble fibre, which helps the gut work more efficiently. Used in remedies alongside a stronger laxative such as senna (see Syrup of Figs, page 46), figs help soothe and prevent stomach pains and griping. The roasted fruit was traditionally mashed and made into a poultice for abscesses in the mouth. Surely worth a try; at least it will taste nice!

GROWS/WHERE TO FIND
→ likes slightly alkaline, free-draining soil
→ place in very sunny position – fan against a south-facing wall
→ restrict roots with rocks or place in a pot to encourage fruit production
→ if grown in pots, overwinter in frost-free conditions
→ fruit usually appears one summer, but doesn't ripen until the following summer
→ buy fresh from greengrocers or supermarkets

Goji Berries
Lycium barbarum

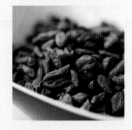

Goji berries sound exotic and are used as a superfood in Chinese medicine, but these glossy scarlet berries also grow wild in southern English hedgerows in autumn, from a plant more commonly known as boxthorn or wolfberry. In recent years, goji berries have become a fashionable cure-all. They are claimed to lower cholesterol, protect the liver, improve eyesight and dizziness, reduce the side effects of chemotherapy, boost circulation and even improve sexual performance in men. What is certain is that the berries contain antioxidants and high levels of vitamin C, which can help various degenerative conditions, and so may help improve memory and eyesight. They also contain certain sugars that are thought to enhance immune function and protect against colds and flu (try Goji Berry and Shiitake Soup, page 111). In other words, these berries are really good for you.

To make Goji Berry Tea, infuse 30 g fresh or dried berries in 500 ml just-boiled water, steep for 10 minutes, then drink (you can eat the berries too).

GROWS/WHERE TO FIND
→ can be difficult to get established, then freely sends out suckers to become invasive
→ likes fertile soil
→ very salt-tolerant
→ found in hedgerows
→ buy dried berries from supermarkets and health food shops

Hops
Humulus lupulus

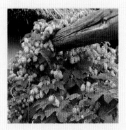

Mild prolonged insomnia can cause real distress, but doctors are rightly reluctant to prescribe sleeping pills. Using hops is a good solution: it's a gentle sedative with none of the addictive or narcotic side effects of commercial sleeping tablets. You can drink it as tea (but add honey, it's bitter), take it as a tincture (see Using Plants, page 34) or use the dried flowers in a sleep-inducing pillow (see recipe on page 121). (Hops are also used in beer, but the sedative effect doesn't survive the brewing process well; it's the alcohol not the hops that make you sleepy.) The yellow flowers, or strobiles, of hops contain bitter acids and essential compounds that are calming and reduce anxiety and nervous excitement generally. They also relieve tension in the gut, thus soothing nervous indigestion. A cup or two of hops tea every day can also help with menopausal symptoms, as it contains oestrogen-boosting compounds.

GROWS/WHERE TO FIND
→ prefers sunny location
→ rampant climber, so provide sturdy supports
→ can overwhelm nearby plants
→ dry flowers

Kiwi Fruit
Actinidia deliciosa

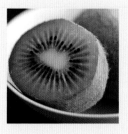

The brown-skinned, green-fleshed, black-seeded kiwi fruit used to be called the Chinese gooseberry and is native to China, where it grows wild. The roots, fruits and leaves of the plant are used in traditional Chinese medicine, but in the West only the fruits are consumed. High in vitamins C and E, potassium, magnesium and copper, the fruit is eaten or processed for use in beauty products to improve skin and hair.

Kiwi fruit have several health benefits: they're thought to have a beneficial effect on heart function, and to decrease the amount of fats in the blood. They also contain lutein, which can improve eye health. They're worth eating regularly for their all-round health benefits, and can also be mashed and made into a variety of homemade facial care products (see Kiwi and Papaya Face Mask, page 136).
NB Kiwi fruit can cause allergies, including skin irritation: if that occurs, discontinue use.

GROWS/WHERE TO FIND
→ vigorous climber, will grow in milder parts of the country
→ likes sun and shelter, eg a south-facing wall
→ needs rich, well-drained soil
→ water and feed in summer
→ male and female plants needed for fruit
→ train as espaliers for best fruit
→ prune 3-year-old stems in winter
→ buy from greengrocers or supermarkets

Lemon
Citrus limon

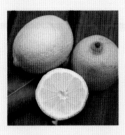

Lemon is one of the most versatile and widely used fruits in the world, primarily as a zesty flavour in cooking. It's high in vitamin C and is often added to cough medicines and pastilles. Applied to the skin, it has antibacterial and astringent effects, which helps to clear up spots and brighten dull or oily skin and hair (see Lemon Jelly Peeling Face Mask, p136). It's also used in many beauty treatments to help with cellulite, though more research is needed in this area. The essential oil, made from lemon zest, has been used to calm, soothe mental fatigue and insomnia, and lighten low mood.

As a hair lightener, add the juice of a lemon to 150 ml water, mix, then apply as a final rinse to hair. Leave on for 5 minutes, then rinse with water.

GROWS/WHERE TO FIND
➜ grow in a pot
➜ likes sun
➜ prefers a sheltered site with free-draining soil
➜ water in summer
➜ fertilize during growing season
➜ place in frost-free situation over winter
➜ will fruit all year round
➜ buy from greengrocers or supermarkets

Milk Thistle Seeds
Silybum marianum

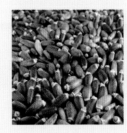

Milk thistle is widely known as a hangover cure, helping the liver when under acute stress and diminishing the knock-on effects, including headaches, skin outbreaks and digestive problems. Milk thistle is powerfully effective at protecting the liver and helping the body to get rid of poisons. For example, taken before eating the death cap mushroom, which contains fatal toxins, it's been shown to give complete protection; it is also effective taken within 48 hours of ingesting the mushroom. In Germany and elsewhere, milk thistle is used to treat chronic hepatitis and cirrhosis of the liver, but seems to be most effective when used as a preventative rather than a long-term solution to liver problems.

To use, grind the seed very finely, take as a tincture or tea (see Using Plants, page 34), or sprinkle 1 tsp on cereal or in a smoothie.

GROWS/WHERE TO FIND
➜ biennial
➜ prefers an open sunny site
➜ self-sows freely – bit of a garden thug
➜ need to grow many plants for useful amount of seed
➜ buy from health food shops

Papaya
Carica papaya

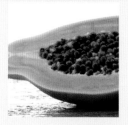

The papaya, or pawpaw, tree grows mostly in tropical countries, but the fruit is popular worldwide. It's delicious eaten on its own but is also useful to aid in the digestion of protein-rich meals – it contains a mixture of enzymes known as papain, which are used commercially as a meat tenderizer. You can buy papaya enzyme tablets for indigestion or eat fresh papaya with or after meals.

Medicinally, papaya is best known for its use in wound healing and skin repair. The green, unripe fruit contains a milky fluid with a high concentration of papain. Applied to skin, it's been shown to help heal burns, slough off dead tissue, improve scar formation, and reduce inflammation and pain. It's used on chronic ulcers and carbuncles, and also for psoriasis, ringworm and other skin infections. Used in face masks and cosmetic skin preparations, it can have a gentle exfoliating effect (see Kiwi Fruit and Papaya Mask, page 136).

NB Do not take tablets during pregnancy.

GROWS/WHERE TO FIND
→ buy papaya enzyme tablets from health food shops
→ buy the fresh fruit from greengrocers or supermarkets

Psyllium Seeds
Plantago psyllium

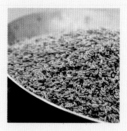

We're used to taking bran as a source of soluble fibre to encourage the digestive process, but psyllium seeds are a better bet, causing less bloating and gas. These tiny, glossy, dark brown seed husks swell up to many times their size to create a gelatinous mass that slowly works through the gut. On the way, it triggers contractions, scrapes the intestinal walls and slows digestion, regulating disorders such as diarrhoea, constipation and diverticulitis.

Even more significantly, psyllium seeds have been found to lower the levels of low-density lipoprotein, or 'bad' cholesterol in the blood, thus helping combat heart disease. They also help lower blood sugar levels by delaying the absorption of sugar, so are useful for diabetics or people at risk of developing diabetes, and may help reduce the risk of colon cancer. Adults can take 20–35 g a day, but do drink lots of water too.

GROWS/WHERE TO FIND
→ annual
→ needs sun
→ grow outdoors from seed sown in late spring
→ buy from health food shops

Red Raspberry Leaf
Rubus idaeus

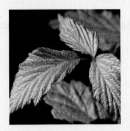

It's the toothed leaves of raspberries, not the delicious summer berries, which are of most benefit in plant remedies. Raspberry leaves were traditionally used during the later stages of pregnancy to ease the birth process (of both humans and animals), make the delivery less painful, and help the uterus get back into shape, but their effectiveness has never been clinically proven. Nowadays, we do not recommend that pregnant women take any remedy that has not been conclusively shown to be safe. However, raspberry leaf tea can be used to lighten heavy periods and help combat menopausal symptoms (see also Sage and Raspberry Leaf Tea on page 94).

For Raspberry Leaf Tea, infuse a handful of fresh raspberry leaves in a mug of just boiled water. Leave for 10 minutes, then strain and drink.

GROWS/WHERE TO FIND
→ likes sun though tolerates partial shade
→ needs moisture-retentive soil
→ net to protect fruit from birds
→ pick leaves throughout growing season

Rosehips
Rosa spp.

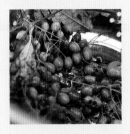

In hedgerows in autumn, there's an abundance of bright scarlet rosehips, the fruit of the wild (or dog) rose. While blackberries are quickly stripped from their stems, few people seem to pick rosehips any more. It's a shame, not least because these tough, hard fruits can be made into a vitamin-rich syrup to keep winter coughs and cold at bay: they contain vitamins A, C and K, plus the B vitamins thiamin, riboflavin and niacin. During World War II, rosehips were collected by children and sold to chemists to be made into syrup. It's easy to make at home: just follow the recipe on page 76. Strain the syrup well; the tiny hairs are irritating and traditionally used as itching powder, dropped by school children down their classmates' backs.

GROWS/WHERE TO FIND
→ wild roses like damp, heavy soils
→ fruit found in hedgerows in September–October
→ take a stepladder when harvesting – they often grow high

VEGETABLES

Artichoke
Cynara scolymus

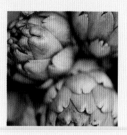

The globe of the artichoke is a culinary delicacy, but the leaves are most beneficial in plant-based medicine, containing a wide range of essential compounds with health-giving benefits for the liver, cardiovascular system and digestive tract. Leaf extract stimulates bile production in the liver, helping with the digestion of fats, and studies have shown it to be effective for treating indigestion and soothing irritable bowel syndrome.

Artichoke has a double effect on cholesterol: it stops it from being produced in the body and contains antioxidants that prevent the oxidation of low-density lipoproteins ('bad' cholesterol). All in all, it has very positive benefits for heart health (see Hawthorn and Artichoke Fruit Leather, page 104).

NB See your GP if you suspect you have abnormally high cholesterol levels. Artichoke should be used as an addition to, not as a substitute for, conventional medical treatment.

To make a tincture, fill a glass jar with fresh, sliced artichoke leaves and cover with vodka, then seal and leave in a dark place for 3 weeks, shaking occasionally. Strain and bottle. Take 30 drops, twice a day.

GROWS/WHERE TO FIND
→ likes fertile, well-drained soil
→ needs a sunny spot
→ grows very tall, so might need supporting
→ watch out for slugs and snails
→ dig manure into surrounding soil in winter
→ protect in cold winters
→ cut young leaves during the growing period

Celery Seeds
Apium graveolens

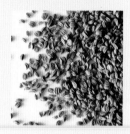

Celery seed was once reputed to be a potent aphrodisiac but nowadays is more usually taken to help with conditions like gout, anxiety and arthritis. It's anti-inflammatory, so decreases swelling in the joints, and is a good diuretic, diluting and flushing gout-causing uric acid more quickly through the system. It also protects against gastric damage caused by painkillers, and has gentle sedative properties, relaxing muscles, calming anxiety and helping sleep. It's probably not worth growing celery just for the seeds (they are tiny and you'd need to devote a large amount of planting space to harvest enough), but they're easily available in health food shops.

Celery Seed Tea: crush 1 tsp seeds and pour over 1 drinking cup freshly boiled water. Infuse for 15 minutes, then strain and drink, up to 3 times a day.

GROWS/WHERE TO FIND
→ likes sun
→ seeds ripen August–October
→ buy as fresh or dried seed, or extract, from health food shops

Chilli, Cayenne Pepper
Capsicum spp.

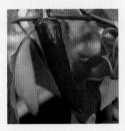

Familiar the world over, chilli comes from the Americas, its strongly pungent flavour adding spice to countless dishes. The constituents responsible for the hot, sometimes fiercely hot, impact of chilli are also those most involved in its many medicinal applications. It can act as an antiseptic, counter-irritant, local analgesic, stimulant and tonic.

When applied to the skin as a counter-irritant, chilli causes a sense of warmth and burning, increasing circulation to the area while desensitising pain. For this reason, chilli is added to lotions, liniments and salves for muscular aches and pains, resulting in better nutrition to – and clearance of waste products from – the tissues involved.

Chilli has antiseptic properties and helps to protect against gastrointestinal infection. It is often added to food in tropical countries to reduce the risk of food poisoning. Used in small quantities, chilli will help strengthen a weak digestive system and stimulate appetite. **To make a peppery oil,** stir 1 part powdered cayenne pepper into 30 parts olive oil and rub into affected area 3 times a day. Do not use on broken skin. (See also Hot Chilli and Mustard Foot Oil, page 70, and Chilli Plasters, page 91.)

GROWS/WHERE TO FIND
→ tender plant
→ grows best in dry soil and full sun
→ easily grown in pots
→ buy from greengrocers or supermarkets

Cucumber
Cucumis sativus

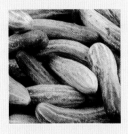

Cucumbers are mostly made up of water (with a few vitamins and minerals), so are gentle diuretics and good for intestinal health. They also slightly lower blood sugar. But they are included here for their excellent use in topical beauty products for the face and skin. As an anti-inflammatory, cucumbers are often the base ingredient in face masks, gels, moisturizers and toners. They have soothing and cooling properties and their high water content means they rehydrate skin, leaving it softer and fuller. (See Lemon Jelly Peeling Face Mask, page 136.)

GROWS/WHERE TO FIND
→ half-hardy
→ likes a humid atmosphere
→ best grown under glass
→ needs large amount of space for huge root run and sprawling habit
→ water and feed regularly
→ support stems
→ buy from greengrocers or supermarkets

Garlic
Allium sativum

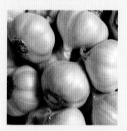

Garlic is a very potent plant: you can smell a big patch of wild garlic, or ramsons (*Allium ursinum*), from metres away. Extracts from the bulbs are natural antiseptics, so are often used in remedies to prevent or combat colds, flu, catarrh and bronchitis, and to reduce nasal congestion. Garlic is also known for its beneficial effects on heart health. Studies show it works by lowering cholesterol levels in the blood, especially of low-density lipoproteins, or 'bad' cholesterol; by slightly lowering blood pressure; and by slowing arterial plaque formation and clots – an effect that seems to be especially marked in women. Overall, garlic may be helpful in the prevention of thrombosis and atherosclerosis (though with any heart condition, herbal remedies should never be taken as a substitute for medical treatment).

Garlic is also coming under the spotlight for its anti-cancer properties. A diet rich in garlic appears to lower the incidence of stomach, colorectal, breast and prostate cancers. Finally, this all-round beneficial plant has significant anti-fungal properties, which make it an excellent external treatment for athlete's foot (see Garlic Talcum Powder and Garlic Foot Bath, pages 52–5), ringworm and other fungal skin diseases.

For a garlic gargle to combat throat infections, pour 200 ml freshly boiled water over 2 peeled and chopped ramsons or garlic bulbs. Leave to steep for 3 hours, then strain and gargle.

Garlic Honey for Coughs: peel and loosely crush 2 heads of garlic, leave exposed to the air for 15 minutes to allow the active ingredient, allicin, to be formed, then crush finely in a mortar and pestle. Mix into a small pot of runny honey and leave overnight. There may be a little 'juice' on the top; just stir in before using. Take 1 tsp for colds, coughs and sore throats as needed.

GROWS/WHERE TO FIND
→ wild garlic in lawns, damp woods
→ can be grown in pots
→ likes sun
→ pick bulbs in autumn
→ buy *A. sativum* from greengrocers or supermarkets

Purslane
Portulaca oleracea

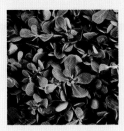

Purslane, an extremely common but pretty weed with fleshy, succulent, lemony-tasting leaves, is well worth cultivating for its unusual health benefits. It is one of the best vegetable sources of vitamin E; glutathione, an antioxidant and detoxifier; and alpha-linolenic acid (ALA), an omega-3 fatty acid we can get only through diet. It's used widely to treat gastric and liver ailments as well as coughs and arthritis. Although few scientific studies have been done on it, purslane is used in herbal remedies and eaten as a salad vegetable across the globe – it was reputedly Gandhi's favourite food. Make it into a tonic as a health booster (see below), juice it with carrots or add a handful of steamed purslane into mashed potatoes.

For a post-viral tonic, gently heat 2 large handfuls purslane leaves and 2 cloves chopped garlic in 500 ml cider vinegar for 20 minutes. Strain and pour into a sterilized bottle. Take 1 tsp twice a day.

GROWS/WHERE TO FIND
→ annual
→ likes full sun
→ not frost-hardy
→ prefers dry soil
→ 2-month growing season
→ cut-and-come-again
→ can be invasive in warm areas

Watercress
Nasturtium officinale

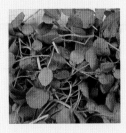

Watercress is one of the most vitamin- and mineral-rich vegetables. It is traditionally given as a remedy for arthritis and upper respiratory tract infections, and as a general spring 'cure', and can also be made into a tonic for the skin and eyes. However, in recent years, it's been investigated for its possible preventative effects against some degenerative diseases, including some cancers. It contains compounds called PEITCs (phenylethyl isothiocyanates) and sulphurophanes (also found in broccoli), which encourage cancer cells to self-destruct as well as building cell defences against carcinogens. Research is still underway, but in the meantime watercress remains a good bet for promoting general all-round health.

As a tea for healthy skin, infuse 1 large handful watercress leaves in 500 ml freshly boiled water and leave for 10 minutes. Strain and drink twice a day.

GROWS/WHERE TO FIND
→ plant seeds in a pot with 6 cm water, half immerse that pot in a second pot, keep water level topped up
→ or grow in shallow trenches in running water or in boggy soil with light shade
→ can give 10 pickings a year
→ buy from greengrocers and supermarkets

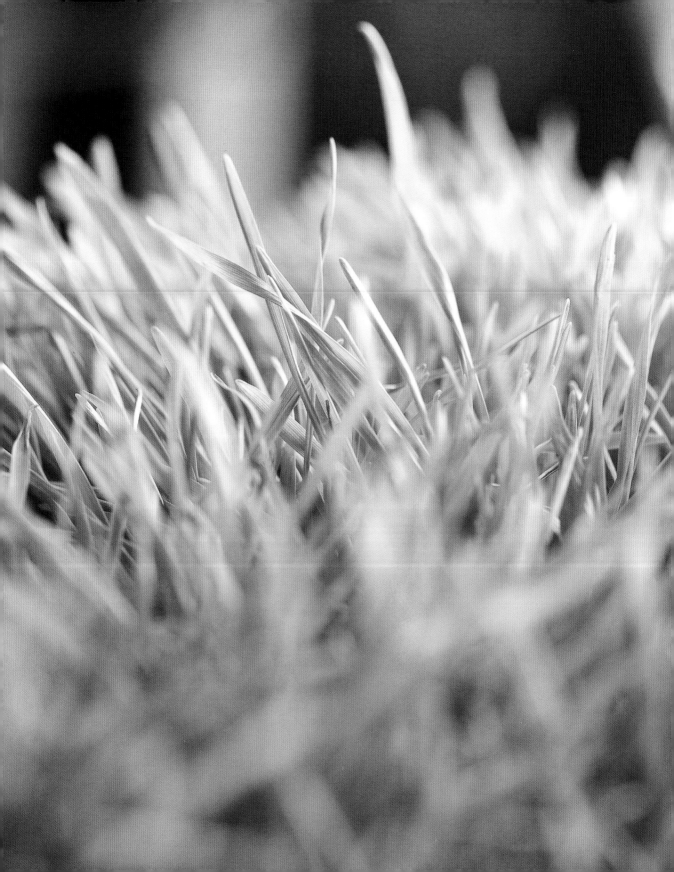

Wheatgrass
Triticum aestivum

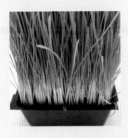

The young, vitamin-rich grass of wheat can easily be grown from seed at home. It improves digestion and has been shown to help in the treatment of some diseases of the colon, including ulcerative colitis. It's hard to digest, so juice before using. Some people enjoy the slightly bitter taste, but if you're not keen, juice with other fruit and vegetables.

GROWS/WHERE TO FIND
→ annual, easily grown from seed
→ sow in rich, well-draining soil in a sunny spot
→ can be grown in trays – soak wheat seeds for 8 hours, sow in small tray with compost/vermiculite mix, water daily
→ harvest when 10 cm high

TREES/SHRUBS

Alder Buckthorn
Rhamnus frangula

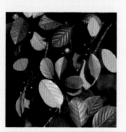

The bark of the alder buckthorn, a small bushy native tree, gives gentle relief from chronic constipation by increasing fluid accumulation in the gut and stimulating the muscular walls of the colon. Cut a young branch (1–2 years old) and strip and discard the outer bark to reveal the papery inner layer below. Always dry the inner bark for a few weeks in a cool dark place before boiling to make decoctions – if used fresh, the active ingredients known as anthraquinones, can make you sick.

For a laxative, simmer 30 g dried bark in 1 litre water for 30 minutes or until halved in volume. Strain, then take 1 tbsp 3 times a day until problem is relieved.

GROWS/WHERE TO FIND
→ found in damp woodland and around fields
→ a good small garden tree, reaching 5 m
→ protect from strong winds

Eucalyptus
Eucalyptus spp.

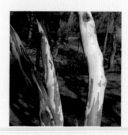

A native of Australia, eucalyptus has long been used by Aborigines as a remedy for colds, sore throats, coughs and bronchitis. The oil from the leaves works as a decongestant and expectorant, and is used widely in over-the-counter cough syrups and sweets. You can make it into a balm (see Pine and Eucalyptus Oil, page 132) for use as a chest rub.

Eucalyptus is an antiseptic used as a topical treatment for wounds and skin infections: apply crushed leaves as a poultice or macerate them in oil and rub in as a liniment. It's also been shown to have a lowering effect on blood sugar levels. Insects dislike the pungent aroma, which makes it a good insect repellent, while herbalists use it as a treatment for bad breath (see Thyme Sweet Breath Spray and Mouthwash, page 41).

For an inhalation for blocked nose and sinuses, pour freshly boiled water on to a handful of crushed eucalyptus leaves in a large bowl. Cool slightly, then put a towel over your head and the bowl, and breathe deeply.

GROWS/WHERE TO FIND
→ found in gardens and woodland
→ likes fertile, well-drained soil
→ needs full sun
→ *Eucalyptus gunnii* is the hardiest species for this country (able to tolerate -15ºC)
→ cut back to manageable size each year (otherwise grows very tall and branches get out of reach)
→ buy oil from pharmacies

Ginkgo
Ginkgo biloba

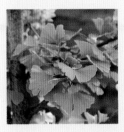

The *ginkgo biloba* or maidenhair tree is thought to have been around for over 225 million years, since the age of the dinosaurs, so it's perhaps fitting that its best-documented benefits are for memory enhancement and the mild-to-moderate dementia that can come with age. The dried leaves contain unique substances that are thought to work by improving circulation to the brain, altering the availability of neuro-transmitters and enzymes which control brain chemistry, and increasing oxygen supply.

Ginkgo has been dubbed the 'wrinklies' wonder drug' because it improves concentration, short-term memory and reaction time in the middle-aged to elderly (see Ginkgo Tea, page 118). It also helps with circulatory disorders including vertigo, cramping pains in the legs and mountain sickness. By opening up the bronchial passages, it helps with asthma and allergic inflammation, and can reduce inhaler use. If you are on prescription medication, speak to your doctor or pharmacist in case taking ginkgo could interfere with its effectiveness or safety.

To improve memory, make an infusion of 30 g dried leaves with 500 ml just boiled water. Leave to steep for 10 minutes and strain, then drink a cup twice a day.

GROWS/WHERE TO FIND
→ slow-growing deciduous conifer
→ full sun
→ pollution-hardy
→ well-drained soil
→ harvest summer leaves, then dry before use

Hawthorn
Crataegus laevigata

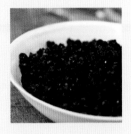

Hawthorn is a common hedgerow plant, and its berries are a known tonic for heart health (see Hawthorn and Artichoke fruit leather recipe, page 104). They contain compounds that help to regulate blood pressure and heart rate and improve blood flow by dilating the arteries. This helps with circulatory problems such as Raynaud's disease and cold extremities. Hawthorn is also thought to reduce anxiety and mood swings, and relieve insomnia.

Hawthorn Syrup: bring 500 g ripe berries and 500 ml water to the boil, then mash and leave overnight. Next day, bring back to the boil, and simmer gently until the berries lose their colour. Strain through muslin, measure the juice into a pan and add the same amount of sugar. Bring to the boil rapidly, then pour into sterilized bottles. Take 1 tsp daily to help maintain a healthy circulation.

NB If you think you have a heart condition, you must also consult your doctor.

GROWS/WHERE TO FIND
→ common hedgerow shrub/tree
→ good as hedging
→ white flowers in spring, red berries in autumn
→ prune only after fruiting

Horse Chestnut
Aesculus hippocastanum

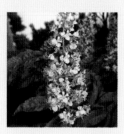

An extract made from conkers, the seeds of the horse chestnut tree, is used as a treatment for varicose veins, piles and swelling in the lower legs. Varicose veins get twisted and 'baggy', damaging the valves that stop blood running backwards, and stopping them working properly. Even more blood then 'pools' in the veins, swelling them. Aescin, the essential compound in extract of horse chestnut, restores the veins' elasticity and improves the flow of blood back to the heart, thus decreasing the risk of clotting and swelling in the lower legs. Horse chesnut can also decrease the likelihood of developing deep-vein thrombosis (DVT), and minimize swelling in the feet and ankles on long flights. Try the Horse Chestnut Gel, page 88.

NB Although commercially prepared horse chestnut extracts are taken orally, do not eat conkers because they are dangerous when untreated.

GROWS/WHERE TO FIND
→ stunning and huge ornamental tree with candelabra flowers
→ found in parks and gardens
→ collect conkers in autumn

Juniper
Juniperus communis

If you suffer from recurrent urinary tract infections, it's a good idea to keep a tincture of juniper berries in your medicine cabinet.

The berries take a couple of years to ripen to a dark purplish black, but as soon as they're ready, pick them and macerate fresh in oil, or use dried and crushed to make teas and tinctures (see Using Plants, page 34). The volatile oil in the berries – used to give gin its traditional bitter flavour – has diuretic and anti-inflammatory properties, which are helpful with both chronic and acute outbreaks of cystitis. Juniper is also used to treat rheumatism, can gently lower both blood pressure and blood sugar levels, and is often made into an antiseptic balm for irritated skin conditions.

NB Avoid during pregnancy. Don't use juniper for longer than 1 month because it can irritate the kidneys.

GROWS/WHERE TO FIND
→ aromatic evergreen conifer
→ found wild throughout Britain, especially on chalky downs
→ likes sun
→ both female and male plants must be grown for fruits
→ collect ripe berries only
→ dry on shelves/trays on greaseproof paper

Lime, Linden
Tilia spp.

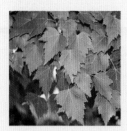

You have to be quick to pick the sweet-smelling blossom of the lime tree: the blooms last for only a couple of weeks in July. They make an excellent dual-purpose tea used primarily to treat feverish colds and flu, but also to calm nervous disorders such as anxiety, irritation and restlessness. The essential compounds lower blood pressure and have a slightly sedative effect, making this a good drink to take a couple of hours before bed. Children like the sweet taste of linden tea, and it can soothe them when they're overactive or feeling anxious.

To make Lime Blossom Tea, put 3 tsp (15 g) dried flowers in 500 ml freshly boiled water. Steep for 10 minutes, then strain. Drink a little throughout the day.

GROWS/WHERE TO FIND
→ easy to grow
→ needs moist soil
→ found in parks and gardens
→ short flowering season
→ collect buds and flowers, dry in a cool, dark place, then store in tight-lidded jars out of sunlight

Neem
Azadirachta indica

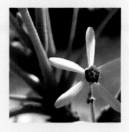

Neem, also known as the Indian lilac, is a large deciduous tree native to India and Southeast Asia. The leaves and seeds are used to treat a variety of ailments, from ulcers and skin diseases to improving digestion and protecting the liver. Like garlic, neem is anti-fungal, antibacterial and antiviral, and also brings down temperature in a fever.

However, in this country neem is used mainly as a treatment for head lice and nits – the eggs of the louse, which become 'cemented' to the hair shaft. Lice are becoming increasingly resistant to conventional over-the-counter treatments, and neem has powerful insecticide properties, providing a natural treatment that is free of organophosphates. Applied to the hair and scalp (see Neem Nit Treatment, page 79), it kills live lice. But, like all treatments for head lice, it needs several re-applications to ensure that all the nits have been dealt with.

GROWS/WHERE TO FIND
→ can grow in a warm conservatory (though it is unlikely to reach a stature where seeds are borne)
→ buy from pharmacies

Pine *Pinus* spp.
and Cedar *Cedrus* spp.

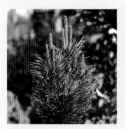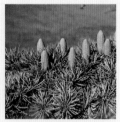

The powerful, 'clean' fragrance and decongestant properties of pine and cedar make them popular additions to many over-the-counter cough and cold remedies. The essential oil is distilled from the needles or collected as resin, and can be used at home in inhalations, made into a balm to warm stiff or painful muscles, or as an antiseptic deodorant (see Pine Spray, page 135) which kills odour-causing germs and covers less pleasant smells.

As a decongestant, try a pine needle steam inhalation. Place 1 handful crushed fresh green pine needles in a bowl, and add 1 litre boiling water. Then inhale the steam and fragrant pine oil by putting your face over the bowl, taking care not to get scalded. Keep the steam in by putting a towel over your head.

GROWS/WHERE TO FIND
→ fast-growing evergreen conifers
→ found in forests, woods, seaside areas
→ like full sun
→ need acid soil
→ inhibit growth of other plants beneath them
→ buy resin (see Resources, page 219)

Slippery Elm
Ulmus rubra

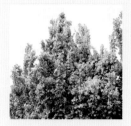

Slippery elm, or red elm, is a US native, though you can find it in parks and gardens throughout Britain. It's a fast grower, reaching 60 m, and takes its unusual name from the pale orangy-yellow inner bark, which is powdered and made into a 'slippery' mucilage by heating with water. The resulting porridge-like gruel is nutrient-rich (George Washington's army was reputed to have survived on it during the brutal winter of 1777–8) but also has a soothing, demulcent effect on the gastrointestinal tract. For this reason, it is recommended for use with ulcers, colitis, constipation and other digestive disorders (flavouring with sugar, honey or spices improves the blandness).

In the United States, slippery elm is added to syrups, pastilles and cough sweets to help with sore throats, viral infections and bronchitis. Coarsely powdered bark can be made into a poultice (see Using Plants page 36) to soothe burns and skin irritations and draw out infection in wounds, spots and boils.

GROWS/WHERE TO FIND
→ likes moist soil
→ needs full sun
→ suffers from Dutch elm disease so is better to buy powdered bark from health food shops

Spruce
Picea spp.

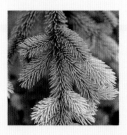

Don't throw away your Christmas tree – it can have healing properties. The traditional Norway spruce, easily grown in this country in pots as well as in the garden, has been found to have anti-microbial properties, limiting the growth of various bacteria. The resin from spruce can be made into a salve (see Using Plants, page 35), and applied to wounds, including spots, ulcers, boils, chronic bed sores and other skin infections. Spruce needles, freshly picked, are also used in Finland to make a soothing inhalation for coughs, colds and flu.

To make an energizing, aromatic bath oil, place a few handfuls of fresh green spruce needles to fill a small, sterilized Kilner jar. Cover with olive oil and leave for 2 weeks, shaking occasionally. Strain and bottle.

GROWS/WHERE TO FIND
→ evergreen conifer
→ found widely in forests and woodland
→ will grow in pots
→ likes damp, acid soil

Tea Tree Oil
Melaleuca alternifolia

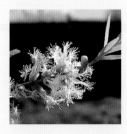

You won't be able to grow a tea tree here (or not outdoors), but the oil is well worth buying and keeping in your medicine cabinet.

It's a natural antiseptic that helps treat bacterial and fungal infections all over the body. The oil, distilled from the leaves and twigs, is marketed as a cure-all and is used in many commercial preparations for acne, skin breakouts, cuts, wounds, dandruff, lice and scabies infestations, bad breath and thrush. Make it into a balm and use for mild-to-moderate acne. It will help reduce pustules and inflammation without the drying and flaking effect caused by many over-the-counter preparations. It's also effective as an anti-fungal lotion or cream for topical use for athlete's foot or nail infections if used regularly for several weeks.

As a mouthwash for oral thrush, dilute 3 drops tea tree oil in ½ drinking cup warm water. Swill around mouth for 60 seconds. Spit out. Do not swallow. Repeat 4 times daily.

NB Do not take tea tree oil internally and keep away from children. Do not use full strength on skin; it can cause contact dermatitis.

GROWS/WHERE TO FIND
→ buy from pharmacies or health food shops
→ can be grown in a cool conservatory, but more as a curiosity than a plant for oil

Top 100 Plants: Trees/Shrubs

Thuja
Thuja occidentalis

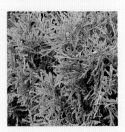

Warts and verrucas are caused by the human papilloma virus. They generally disappear by themselves, but this can take a long time – 2 years or more is normal. They're contagious by touch, so it's a good idea to speed up the process if you can. The leaves and branch ends of thuja, an evergreen conifer that grows widely in Britain, have been widely used traditionally to treat warts and verrucas. It seems to work most successfully on small to medium-sized warts – the large, spreading cauliflower-type warts are harder to treat.

You can also harvest and dry the leaves/branch tips, then make them into a tincture, oil or balm (see Using Plants, page 34) to use directly on skin to soothe rheumatic pains, neuralgia and sore muscles.
NB The essential compound is called thujone, which is toxic when taken internally in large doses. Thuja also stimulates contractions of the womb and encourages menstruation, so should not be taken internally by pregnant women.

GROWS/WHERE TO FIND
→ easy-to-grow evergreen conifer
→ likes moist, deep soil
→ grow in a sheltered site
→ needs full sun

Uva-ursi
Arctostaphylos uva-ursi

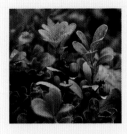

The leaves of uva-ursi or bearberry, a small evergreen shrub, are used to treat urinary tract infections, including cystitis and inflammation of the urethra. It is often sold in a mixture of herbs as a bladder and kidney tonic tea. Used with dandelion in one trial, uva-ursi was shown to have a signficant effect on recurrent cystitis and has also been used to treat frequent and painful urination.

GROWS/WHERE TO FIND
→ small evergreen shrub
→ prefers damp, acid soil
→ harvest green leaves in early autumn, then dry

Willow Bark
Salix alba spp.

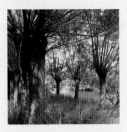

If you've ever taken aspirin, you'll have experienced the painkilling effect of salicin, the active compound in willow, which is converted in the body to the same compound as aspirin (salicylic acid). In fact, chewing on a piece of willow bark has been a well-known headache remedy for hundreds of years. In trials, the bark has also been shown to have significant success in relieving painful inflammatory conditions such as osteoarthritis, back pain and rheumatism.

It's best to harvest the bark in the spring. You can use any willow, though it's worth knowing that the common white willow (*Salix alba*) is less potent than crack willow (*S. fragilis*), purple willow (*S. purpurea*) or violet willow (*S. daphnoides*). With a sharp knife, strip off lengths from young branches, being careful to take only a little bark from each one. You can dry the bark for decoctions, or make it into a tincture (see Using Plants, page 34). Use as you would aspirin, for pain relief from headaches, period pains, sports injuries, backache, muscle aches and arthritis. It also brings down high temperatures, so can be used for relief from colds and flu.

Although willow bark is slower to act than popping an aspirin, the effect is longer lasting. It's also less likely than aspirin to cause gastric problems and internal bleeding, so makes a good substitute for people with sensitive stomachs. NB Be aware that willow bark does not have the same blood-thinning effects as aspirin. Do not take during pregnancy or when breastfeeding.

GROWS/WHERE TO FIND
→ deciduous tree, often growing along riversides and in hedgerows
→ likes wet/damp soil in sun
→ roots are invasive, so don't grow near buildings

Witch Hazel
Hamamelis virginiana

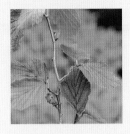

If you want one top performer in your medicine cabinet for everyday family ailments, make it a bottle of witch hazel. The extract of this winter-flowering shrub is the first port of call for bruises, sprains, burns, spots, boils and general skin irritations, and can help reduce bleeding when applied topically to wounds. It's highly regarded as an astringent to contract the swelling of varicose veins and piles, and is a successful antiviral in the treatment of cold sores (*Herpes simplex*). It can also be used as a soother and anti-inflammatory for sore throats and laryngitis.

You can buy ointments and lotions made from the leaves, and the twigs are steam-distilled to make extract of witch hazel BP for normal household use. To make a gel to help with the treatment of spots, see page 60.
To make a witch hazel gargle for sore throats, mix ½ tsp leaves and ½ tsp bark with 500 ml freshly boiled water. Leave, covered, for 1 hour. Strain and use to gargle 3 times a day.

GROWS/WHERE TO FIND
→ hardy but slow-growing deciduous shrub
→ likes damp soil and sun
→ sweet-smelling winter flowers
→ use leaves in spring and summer
→ buy the extract from pharmacies

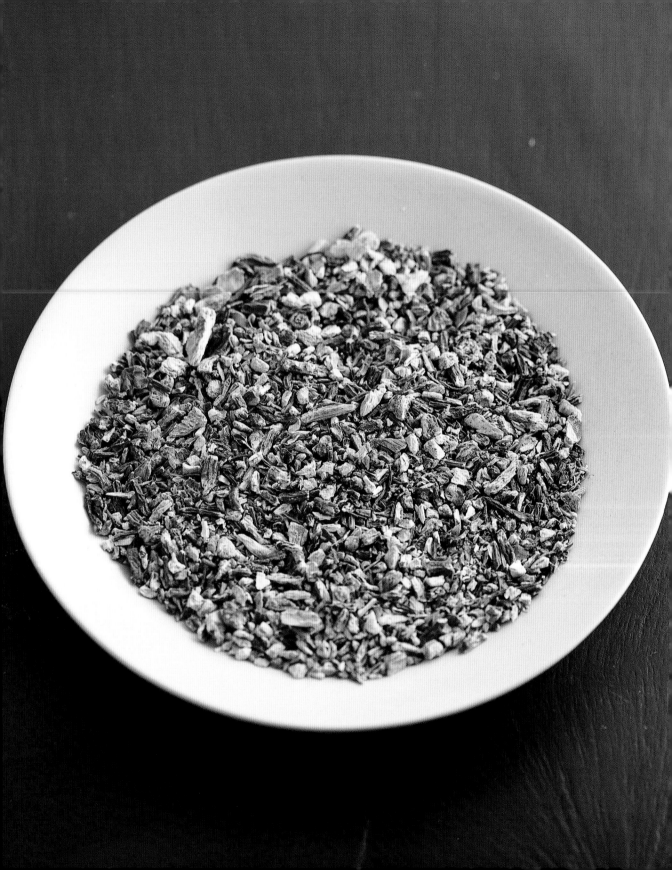

ROOTS

Angelica Root
Angelica archangelica

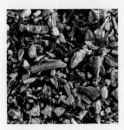 If you know of angelica only as candied green cake decorations or as a flavouring in liqueurs, think again. This common but statuesque plant has many medicinal uses, and is especially good in the treatment of indigestion, easing griping pains and getting rid of wind. It's also used as an appetite-stimulator. It's anti-inflammatory and expectorant, helpful in making coughs, catarrh and nasal congestion looser and more productive – you can make it into a honey or drink as a decoction (see Using Plants, page 34). It also powers heat round to cold extremities: it has a reputation as a 'warming' herb, increasing blood flow to the arms and lower legs.

Angelica grows so prolifically along country roadsides and hedgerows that you can easily pick enough without planting it in the garden, but if you do so, be careful to identify it correctly as the many members of parsley family look very similar. The roots are the most powerful part, though flowers, stalks and seeds can be used too. Harvest roots in the autumn of their first year of growth, then slice in half and dry before using.

To soothe windy tummies, simmer 30 g chopped dried angelica root in a pan with 1 litre water for 20 minutes (until reduced by half). Strain and drink 3 times a day. (See also Angelica Tummy Soother, page 44.)

GROWS/WHERE TO FIND
→ biennial, or to keep as a perennial, remove the flowerheads to stop seed setting
→ likes damp soil
→ grows wild
→ grows to 2 m
→ needs staking
→ blooms June–July
→ harvest roots in autumn

Black Cohosh
Actaea racemosa

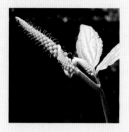

Black cohosh, the bugbane plant, is often taken to relieve the symptoms of menopause, including hot flushes, night sweats, depression and anxiety. It's supposed to give the benefits of oestrogen replacement by balancing the hormones, without any of the unwanted side effects of taking oestrogens. It's also used to regulate periods and soothe rheumatic and other inflammatory conditions.

Although the menopause-easing effects of black cohosh have had positive reports from the Continent over many years, scientific studies have not yet replicated the effects, so more work needs to be done. In the meantime, it may be worth seeing if black cohosh works for you. The plant is easy to grow in gardens, and the root should be dried before making into decoctions or tinctures (see Using Plants, page 34).

NB Don't use during pregnancy and don't take for more than 6 months. Blue cohosh is not from the same plant family.

GROWS/WHERE TO FIND
→ likes moist soil in light shade
→ nutrient-greedy, so inhibits plants around it
→ divide clumps when they get large
→ harvest roots in autumn
→ rinse roots, then leave for several weeks to dry
→ buy extract from health food shops

Chicory
Cichorium intybus

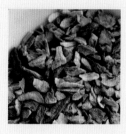

Wild chicory is rather like dandelion: a weed that grows prolifically with sky-blue, dandelion-like flowers, narrow leaves and a milky tap root. Both leaves and root are harvested for herbal remedies. Made into a decoction, the roots have traditionally been used for gout and rheumatism, perhaps due to chicory's diuretic properties, and also as a liver protectant.

Chicory seems to provide a broad spectrum of moderate health benefits: mildly laxative, it's anti-inflammatory, and can lower blood sugar and cholesterol. Although not well known here, it's a very popular remedy in Turkey and the Near East, and is used in Germany as a bitter herb to treat indigestion and increase appetite. As you can grow or pick it easily in the wild, it's definitely worth adding to the herbal cabinet. Chicons, the chicory hearts eaten in salads, can be forced from the roots from November onwards.

For indigestion, boil 1 large handful chopped chicory root in 500 ml water for 10–15 minutes. Strain and drink to soothe heartburn and acid reflux.

GROWS/WHERE TO FIND
→ likes well-drained alkaline soil
→ sow seeds late spring
→ needs deep soil for root development
→ use leaves before it seeds
→ harvest roots in second year, dry for 2 weeks before using

Cleavers
Galium aparine

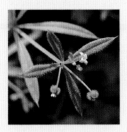

Also known as bedstraw, beggar lice, bur head, catch weed, cling rascal, goose grass, scratch weed and sticky willy, this is a plant with a history. In medieval times, cleavers was used as a cure-all, but today it is better known as a diuretic, which helps with swollen lymph glands, recurrent cystitis and other irritations of the urinary tract. The leaves can be infused to drink as a tea (see Using Plants, page 34), but remember to wear gloves when picking – the stems are covered with short, sharp prickles and the burrs (seeds) stick to everything. Cleavers can also be made into a skin-softening balm.

To soothe nettle stings, sores and skin inflammations, pick a handful of leaves (use gloves), crush with a mortar and pestle, and apply directly to the spot, rubbing gently.

For a spring tonic, pick equal amounts of cleavers, dandelion roots and leaves, nettle ends and burdock roots, then wash and place tightly in a Kilner jar. Pour over enough vodka to cover. Leave for 4 weeks, shaking occasionally. Squeeze by hand the mixture through muslin, then bottle. Take 1 tsp, 1–2 times a day.

GROWS/WHERE TO FIND
→ annual
→ grows easily in most situations
→ prefers alkaline soil
→ pick from hedgerows or banks rather than introducing to your garden

Dandelion
Taraxacum officinale

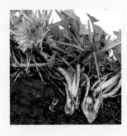

Next time you weed the garden, don't throw out the handfuls of dandelions you've doubtless pulled up. Instead, use them to make plant remedies. Although the root is most often used medicinally, every bit of the dandelion can be used: the flowers in soothing oils; the leaves in infusions (and salads – try them; they're bitter but tasty); the roots as decoctions and tinctures (see Using Plants, page 34). Dandelion is a gentle diuretic and is used traditionally for urinary disorders and poor digestion. Most diuretics leach potassium from the body, but dandelion, apart from being mild, is very high in potassium and other minerals and vitamins, so it also makes a good all-round health tonic.

To make Dandelion Flower Bath Oil, pick enough fresh flowerheads to fill a small Kilner jar. Pour olive oil over to cover, pushing a knife around inside to get rid of any air pockets. Cover and leave on a sunny windowsill for 2 weeks, or until the flowers have lost their colour. Strain, then pour into a sterilized bottle. Soothes muscles and joints.

GROWS/WHERE TO FIND
→ perennial
→ abundant in lawns, fields, banks
→ pick flowers throughout growing season
→ pick roots in autumn and dry before use

Echinacea
Echinacea spp.

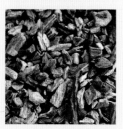

There's not much around that can help treat the common cold, except echinacea. Take it as soon as you feel the signs of infection coming on – many studies show it lessens the severity and duration of colds and flu. Try the ice lolly recipe, page 100, and throat spray on page 116.

No one quite knows how echinacea works, though it's thought to stimulate the immune system and localize the infection, slowing its spread through the body. It has best results when used over an 8–10 day period after infection, so don't bother taking it as a long-term prophylatic to prevent colds coming on – it won't work. As an antibacterial, echinacea is also used in skin preparations to heal wounds, septicaemia, boils and carbuncles. NB When growing in a garden, plant *E. angustifolia*: the roots contain more of the known active constituents than the other two main species, *E. purpurea* and *E. pallida*.

GROWS/WHERE TO FIND
→ perennial
→ likes sun
→ needs rich, sandy soil
→ grow in airy, open site (echinacea is prone to mildews)
→ harvest roots and rhizomes in autumn
→ dry before using in decoctions or tinctures
→ buy extract from pharmacies

Ginger
Zingiber officinale

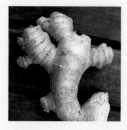

Ginger is one of the most versatile culinary spices, used the world over in both sweet and savoury foods and drinks. But its primary use in remedies is an anti-emetic to prevent or control all kinds of nausea, including motion sickness, morning sickness and vertigo. It's safe enough in moderate doses to be used by both pregnant women and children (see Crystallized Ginger, page 97).

The fresh 'roots' – actually rhizomes or underground stems – contain essential compounds called gingerols. When dried or extracted, these become shogaols, much hotter to the taste, and also twice as potent. These seem to have a blocking effect on certain types of serotonin receptors involved in sickness, suppressing gastric acid production and reducing vomiting. This has a soothing effect on the digestive tract and quells stomach disorders like dyspepsia.

Ginger also has a warming effect on the body, and makes a good tea to take on a winter afternoon. It's also thought to be helpful as an anti-inflammatory for arthritic joints and rheumatic pains.

For a warming ginger tea, peel and chop
5 cm root, then pour a cupful of boiling water
over and leave for 8 minutes. If you like, add
honey or a squeeze of fresh lemon juice to taste.

GROWS/WHERE TO FIND

→ can be grown at home – choose a budding
rhizome (with a little green 'horn')

→ suspend over water with cocktail sticks until
roots form, then pot on; or plant 10–20 cm deep
in potting compost

→ keep warm and moist

→ likes light shade

→ no direct sunlight

→ not frost-tolerant; keep indoors in winter

→ harvest rhizomes when 1 year old

→ buy from greengrocers or supermarkets

Horseradish
Armoracia rusticana

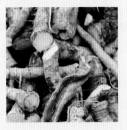

This pungent,
eye-watering root
is traditionally
served as a relish
with roast beef.
Like mustard,
it is bitingly hot
and has a stimulating effect on the body. It's
very easy to grow – indeed it has thuggish
tendencies in the garden – with docklike leaves
and yellowy-white roots. The edible roots can
be made into a balm (see Using Plants, page 35)
to rub on to aching muscles or stiff joints,
encouraging blood to rush to the area.
Horseradish stimulates the digestive system,
encourages sweating and clears the nasal
passages, and can be made into a tincture for
use for colds, flu and coughs.

GROWS/WHERE TO FIND

→ perennial

→ grow in a large container

→ very invasive roots

→ harvest roots in autumn

Liquorice
Glycyrrhiza glabra

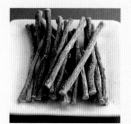

Liquorice root is the single most popular ingredient in Chinese medicine, prescribed in many herb mixtures as a harmonizer. In Britain, it's a common flavouring in sweets, most famously chewy Pontefract cakes, made in the Yorkshire town since the 18th century. Liquorice is known to loosen congestion in respiratory tract infections, and has a long history of use for soothing coughs, colds, bronchitis and sore throats (see Marshmallow and Liquorice Cough Syrup, page 103). It's also anti-inflammatory and has slight anti-allergenic properties, and is used by some herbalists to help with asthma.

It has anti-ulcer effects too, so if you suffer from gastric ulcers, try taking a tincture or decoction of liquorice, or make it into a gargle for mouth ulcers. As a soother or demulcent, it's used for a wide range of stomach disorders, from indigestion to constipation and bowel spasm. In Japan, studies have also shown it to protect the liver and have benefits for chronic hepatitis.

NB Take only small amounts of liquorice (not more than 20 g a day) for up to 4 weeks.

GROWS/WHERE TO FIND
→ perennial
→ likes protected site in sun
→ needs deep root run
→ grows to 1.4 m, so best to stake
→ harvest roots from 3–4-year-old plants

Marshmallow
Althaea officinale

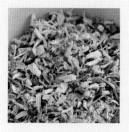

Marshmallow is essentially a gentle soother. The roots and leaves contain a high level of mucilage, a gelatinous substance that can soothe and reduce inflammation in the respiratory, urinary and digestive tracts. Marshmallow is well known as an expectorant and cough-preventer, often found in cough sweets and syrups for sore throats and bronchial complaints. Indeed, the French have used it for centuries in soft cough lozenges called pâte de guimauve; these bear no relation to the gelatinous marshmallows we eat as sweets today, which contain little if any marshmallow root. As a stomach soother, marshmallow is gentle enough to be used by all ages, especially for peptic ulcers and gastric inflammation. Applied externally as a poultice or balm, it soothes, soften and heals, reducing inflammation in infected skin complaints such as ulcers, boils and abscesses.

GROWS/WHERE TO FIND
→ perennial
→ likes sun
→ prefers moist soil
→ needs support at full height
→ harvest roots from plants 3–5 years old

Turmeric
Curcuma longa

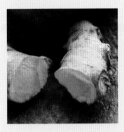

This dark yellow curry plant is widely regarded in India as a tonic for digestive and liver disorders and as a wound healer. It's the active ingredient in 'golden milk', an Ayurvedic cure-all.

Turmeric is increasingly being used by herbalists here as an anti-inflammatory for the stiffness and pain of arthritic joints and for skin diseases, either applied externally as a paste or ointment or taken internally by tincture or decoction. The underground stems, or rhizomes, contain essential compounds that have been shown experimentally to reduce inflammation and also to have a liver-protective effect. However, turmeric is hard to grow in Britain: it is much easier to use dried powdered root instead.

To make a paste for wounds, put 30 g dried turmeric powder in a pan with 150 ml water and simmer to a thick paste. Place gauze on affected area and apply the paste for a few minutes, 3 times a day.

To make Golden Milk, put 200 ml milk, ½ tsp turmeric paste (see above), 1 tsp almond oil and honey (to taste) in a pan. Heat to just below boiling point. Then whizz in a blender to froth (adding fruit such as bananas and berries, if liked). Drink as a health-giving smoothie.

GROWS/WHERE TO FIND
→ native to southern India
→ tender, tropical plant; grow in pots under glass
→ likes light shade
→ keep dry over winter months
→ buy as dried powder from supermarkets

Valerian
Valeriana officinalis

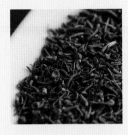

This statuesque plant is well worth planting at the back of borders for its pink-white flowers and divided leaves. And if you're an insomniac or poor sleeper, there's even more cause. Valerian is a natural, effective tranquillizer, reducing the time taken to fall asleep and improving the quality of sleep during the night (see Valerian Hot Chocolate, page 123). It's very safe, with no adverse effects when taken with alcohol, and without any next-day 'hangover' problems – sleepiness, lack of concentration or alertness. The sedative effect also calms anxiety, hyperactivity, nervous tension and irritations arising from stress, and can be useful in the treatment of generalized anxiety disorder (GAD).

Make the roots into decoctions and tinctures for daily use (see Using Plants, page 34). Valerian is more effective when taken over a period of 4 weeks and does not have dependency or withdrawal problems. But be warned: it doesn't smell nice.

GROWS/WHERE TO FIND
→ easy to grow
→ likes sun or semi-shade
→ produces more roots if not allowed to flower
→ protect from cats, which like to roll in it
→ harvest roots in autumn from 2-year-old plants

HERBS

Centaury
Centaurium erythraea

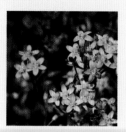

Centaury grows prolifically in chalky meadows and grassy banks, but it's an easy plant to overlook: the pink starlike flowers are in evidence from June to September, but they open for only a few hours a day when the weather is sunny. Centaury is from the same family as gentian, and it has many of the same properties as that alpine herb. Once upon a time, it was called 'bitterwort' and it is *very* bitter, being used as a flavouring in vermouths and other alcoholic aperitifs. It is traditionally used for disorders of the upper digestive tract such as heartburn and indigestion, as well as a tonic for liver and gall bladder complaints. Taken before meals, it's thought to stimulate the appetite.

Pick the whole plant during the flowering season and dry before making into tinctures or infusions (see Using Plants, page 34). Sip slowly to allow the bitter compounds to encourage activity in the digestive tract. Freshly crushed leaves can also be used as a poultice for sores and irritations on the skin.

To settle the stomach, take 15 g dried herb and infuse for 10 minutes in 500 ml freshly boiled water. Strain, and add honey to taste (it will be bitter). Sip slowly.

GROWS/WHERE TO FIND
→ biennial meadow plant
→ difficult to grow in gardens
→ plant in wildflower meadow
→ likes full sun
→ harvest whole plant and dry for later use

Dill
Anethum graveolens

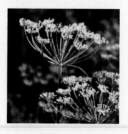

The feathery, flavoursome leaves of dill are known worldwide as a culinary herb, but the seeds are more commonly harvested for use in herbal remedies. Dill seed has a mild effect and pleasant flavour and is used to help calm digestive disorders, especially those involving abdominal gas or intestinal spasms. Crushed, then made into a decoction, the seeds can help ease griping pains and expel wind. Dill seed was traditionally used in gripe water as a treatment for colic in infants. Chewing dried dill seeds on a regular basis is thought to alleviate bad breath.

To dry dill seeds: when the seeds are ripe and brown on the stem (usually around August), cut the stems off, bunch a few together and tie inside a paper bag. Hang upside down in a dry, cool, well-ventilated place for a couple of weeks. Shake, and the seeds will drop out into the bag. Store them in an airtight container.

To make a dill seed tea, steep 30 g dried seeds in 500 ml freshly boiled water. Leave for 10 minutes and strain, then drink as a stomach soother after meals.

GROWS/WHERE TO FIND
→ annual
→ easy to grow from seed
→ 2 weeks germination (if warm)
→ self-sows abundantly
→ inhibits the growth of carrots
→ seeds ripen July–August

Eyebright
Euphrasia officinalis

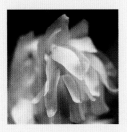

The flowers of eyebright are extremely striking – white with dark purple lines and a central yellow spot. In fact, they look rather like eyes. From the 16th century onwards, the idea that a plant's appearance offered clues to its medicinal use was very popular – a concept called the Doctrine of Signatures. This is perhaps when eyebright started to be used to treat all kinds of eye problems. Little research has been done into eyebright's efficacy, but one recent study showed positive results for use in the treatment of conjunctivitis. Certainly, eyebright has astringent properties, contracting and soothing inflamed tissues, which can help with many eye conditions. You can make it into an eye wash (see page 147) or bathe eyes with a soothing eyebright compress. You can even drink it as a tea (see Using Plants, page 34): it's thought to soothe the upper respiratory tract and to be good as a lung tonic too.

GROWS/WHERE TO FIND
→ annual
→ found in meadows
→ likes chalk soils
→ needs full sun
→ grow from seed in moist soil in late spring
→ semi-parasitic – its roots feed off neighbouring plants' roots
→ harvest leaves and flowers while plant is in bloom

Fenugreek
Trigonella foenum-graecum

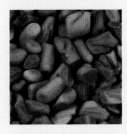

Fenugreek is a native of North Africa and the Mediterranean region and today is widely cultivated in India for use in curry powders, pickles, chutneys and sauces. The nutritious seeds have a distinctive tang described as somewhere between celery and maple syrup, and are also used in sweet dishes from the Middle East, including some recipes for halva. The seeds contain a high percentage of mucilaginous fibre, which accounts for its traditional use as a digestive aid for dyspepsia, diarrhoea and gas. It soothes and relaxes intestinal passageways and is sometimes used to treat gastric ulcers. Recently, fenugreek has also been shown to reduce both 'bad' cholesterol (low-density lipoprotein) and blood sugar levels in people with mild, non-insulin-dependent diabetes.

For glossy hair, crush a small handful of fenugreek seeds in a mortar and pestle, then mix with 3 tbsp natural yoghurt. Apply as a conditioner, leaving on the hair for at least 5 minutes. Rinse out.

To make a stomach-soothing tea, boil 30 g dried fenugreek seeds in 500 ml water for 10 minutes. Strain and sweeten with honey or sugar. NB Don't use during pregnancy because it can stimulate uterine activity.

GROWS/WHERE TO FIND
→ annual
→ can be grown in the United Kingdom, but only in sheltered sites in full sunshine
→ will take 4–5 months for seed to ripen
→ buy from health food shops

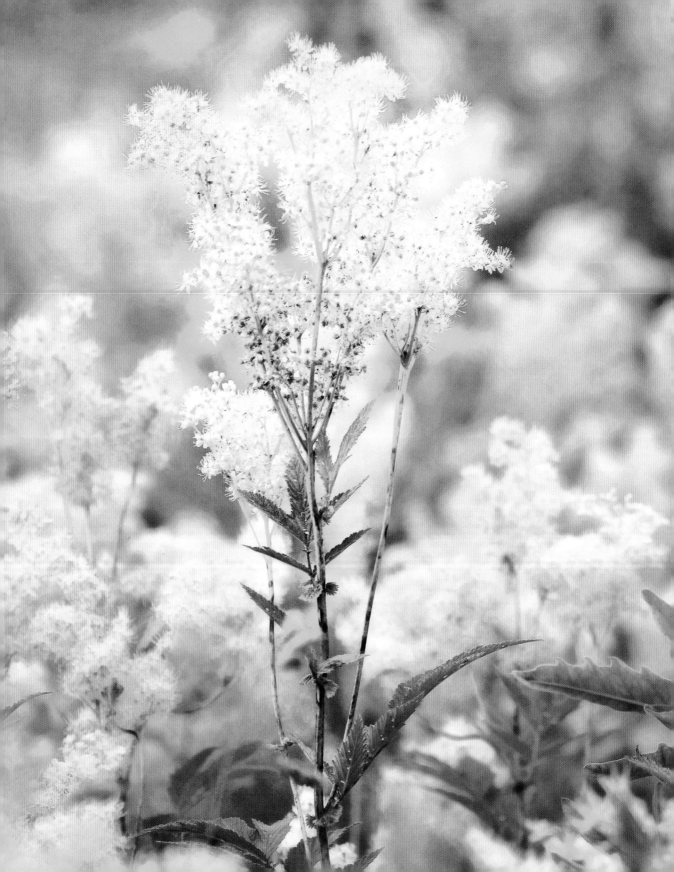

Lemon Balm
Melissa officinalis

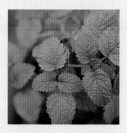

An extremely useful plant to colonize dry, dusty areas of the garden where nothing else will grow. The smell is an added bonus – crush a couple of leaves whenever you walk past to release the tangy lemon aroma. Lemon balm has traditionally been used to soothe nervous tension, relieve anxiety and promote good sleep. It's also been shown to inhibit the growth of the herpes virus, which causes cold sores (see Lemon Balm Lip Salve, page 108).

To calm anxiety and improve sleep: make an infusion using 30 g fresh leaves, crushed, in 500 ml freshly boiled water. Leave, covered, for 10 minutes, then strain and pour into a bath taken before bed.

GROWS/WHERE TO FIND
→ grows well in any site or soil
→ prolifically self-seeding
→ can become a garden nuisance
→ cut back hard after flowering to produce fresh crop of leaves
→ attracts bees

Meadowsweet
Filipendula ulmaria

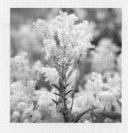

Walking in marshlands or wet woodlands in summer, you'll see the creamy, billowing flowers and tall, reddish stalks of meadowsweet everywhere, like plumes of candy floss on sticks. Harvest the flowering tops on a sunny day, dry them for a couple of weeks, then make into a tea or tincture (see Using Plants, page 34). Meadowsweet is useful in the treatment of acid stomach disorders such as heartburn, indigestion and gastritis, its antacid and inflammatory properties calming and soothing the stomach.

Meadowsweet, like willow bark, also contains the painkilling substance from which aspirin was developed, and has a history of use as an analgesic for headaches. Taken as a tea or applied externally as a compress, it can also help to relieve the inflammation and pain of joint problems like rheumatism, arthritis and gout.

For a compress for sore joints, soak a thin cotton cloth in a strong, hot infusion of meadowsweet tea. Apply to the joints, leave for a couple of minutes, then refresh.

GROWS/WHERE TO FIND
→ perennial
→ likes damp, even wet, soil
→ needs full sun
→ ditches and marshes
→ grow in a marshy patch of meadow or lawn
→ dry the flowering tops

Parsley
Petroselinum crispum

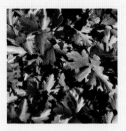

Parsley is one of the most widely grown herbs in this country, but despite being extremely nutritious – high in protein, iron, potassium, magnesium, and vitamins A, some Bs and C – it's more often used as a garnish than a foodstuff. It has a strong flavour eaten raw or cooked, but is more palatable if made into teas or tinctures (see Using Plants, page 34). Traditionally, all parts of the plant are considered to have medicinal properties, especially the root and seed, which have anti-inflammatory properties. Parsley has been used as a diuretic for water retention and mild kidney and bladder disorders – but is not recommended if you have acute or serious kidney problems. It stimulates the kidneys, has an antiseptic effect on the urinary system, and relieves spasms and wind in the digestive tract. It's also helpful with anaemia, improving iron intake and absorption. Chewing fresh parsley leaves can help sweeten breath by masking other strong odours – especially useful after a garlic-laden meal.

As an insect repellent, the juice from the leaves can be rubbed into exposed areas of skin.

NB Avoid excessive use of parsley seed and root during pregnancy.

GROWS/WHERE TO FIND
→ biennial
→ likes a sunny site
→ easy to grow from seed in the sun
→ grow in pots
→ cut-and-cut-again plant
→ harvest leaves before flowering
→ use fresh
→ buy from greengrocers or supermarkets

Peppermint
Mentha x piperita

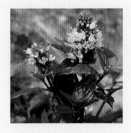

Peppermint has one very unusual effect: at first, it's hot to the tongue (the pepper) and then refreshingly cool (the mint), hence its name. This hybrid between spearmint and water mint is widely used as a flavouring in food, sweets, cosmetics, toothpastes and bath products, giving a clean, sharp taste or smell. Peppermint leaves have been used for hundreds of years to soothe digestive problems, including bloating and dyspepsia (see Angelica Tummy Soother, page 44, and 'Four Winds' Tea, page 49). Recent studies have shown that it has a very positive effect on the symptoms of irritable bowel syndrome, relieving pain and reducing muscle spasms and flatulence. It also relaxes the gullet, which helps get rid of gas in the upper digestive system through belching.

Peppermint oil is good for tension headaches too. Rubbing a dilute solution of essential oil (not more than 1 part oil to 10 parts water) into the temples and forehead can bring significant relief from headache pain. Peppermint can be found in many over-the-counter cough and cold remedies to relieve nasal congestion and catarrh.

NB Don't use the essential oil for infants, either internally or externally.

Relieve nasal congestion with a peppermint inhalation. Put 30 g fresh leaves or 3 drops essential oil in a bowl of freshly boiled water. Leave to cool slightly. Place a towel over your head and the bowl and inhale for a few minutes, being careful to avoid scalding.

GROWS/WHERE TO FIND

→ hardy perennial
→ likes moist soil
→ prefers partial shade
→ creeping roots
→ spreads rapidly
→ grow in pots
→ cut-and-come-again plant
→ harvest leaves throughout growing season
→ buy essential oil from pharmacies

Plantain
Plantago major

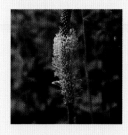

Lawns look bare and rather unnatural without the lush leaves of a few plantain plants pushing up through them. You'll find this weed on almost every path when you go walking, but that's useful because plantain is one of the best remedies for insect bites and stings. In fact, rubbed on to skin after a nettle sting, plantain – especially ribwort or *Plantago lanceolata* – is thought to be more effective than dock leaves. Plantain decreases swelling and is a natural antihistamine, and a simple poultice of fresh green leaves will help with wound healing, bleeding, infections and other skin conditions. Make a plantain balm to take with you on trips to the countryside (see also Plantain Cream, page 58). Alternatively, use it as a decongestant and expectorant to help make coughs and sinusitis more productive. You can drink it as a tea (see Using Plants, page 34) to soothe these and other infections of the upper respiratory tract.

GROWS/WHERE TO FIND

→ in lawns or footpaths
→ weed
→ likes full sun
→ pick leaves at any time and use fresh
→ make tinctures from summer-picked leaves
→ can be dried for use as tea

Rosemary
Rosmarinus officinalis

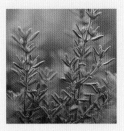

Rosemary is one of the most versatile culinary herbs, an evergreen with a deliciously aromatic flavour often used with fatty meats like lamb. It's easy to grow in the garden, and you can cut off a sprig whenever it's needed, summer or winter. Rosemary is traditionally known as the 'herb of remembrance', and studies show there may be some truth in that claim. It contains compounds that relax the muscles of the digestive tract and can increase the effects of essential enzymes in the brain, thus helping to improve concentration and memory (see Rosemary Wine, page 126).

This stimulating plant can lighten mood and help overcome nervous exhaustion, anxiety and mild depression. Just smelling it can make you feel better, but to cheer yourself up, drink a cup of rosemary tea or take it as a tincture (see Using Plants, page 34). You'll often see rosemary used in shampoos and conditioners for dandruff and thinning hair, including alopecia, as well as a gargle to sweeten breath. **For a breath freshener,** pour 500 ml freshly boiled water over 30 g dried rosemary, then cover and steep for 30 minutes. Strain and gargle several times a day. Store, covered, in a sterilized container in the refrigerator.

GROWS/WHERE TO FIND

→ evergreen shrub
→ needs full sun
→ likes poor soil
→ winter-flowering
→ easy to grow
→ prune in spring after flowering
→ in small gardens, try low-growing 'Prostratus Group'
→ buy fresh herb from supermarkets and essential oil from pharmacies

Sage
Salvia officinalis

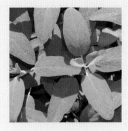

The soft, downy, grey-green leaves of sage don't look as if they pack a big punch. But this aromatic herb has been used in cooking and remedies for over 2000 years in its native Greece and Italy. It's considered something of a cure-all: like rosemary, it has a reputation as a memory enhancer, diuretic and digestive aid, and can even help to keep teeth clean (try Sage and Sea-salt Toothpowder, page 151). But perhaps it's best known for treating colds, coughs and loosening mucus in the upper respiratory tract. You can use it as a throat-soothing honey (see Sage Honey, page 117) or as a gargle infusion for sore throats, tonsillitis, inflamed gums and mouth ulcers.

Sage is used to help ease women through hot flushes, night sweats and other symptoms of menopause (try Sage and Raspberry Leaf Tea, page 94), as well as to reduce lactation. NB Don't take sage during pregnancy or when breastfeeding.

GROWS/WHERE TO FIND

→ evergreen perennial
→ hates wet soil, especially in winter
→ likes sun
→ clip back each year to prevent woodiness
→ harvest leaves just before plants bloom for drying
→ buy fresh herb from supermarkets

Skullcap
Scutellaria lateriflora

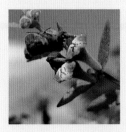

Skullcap is also known as hoodwort, Quaker bonnet and helmet flower – its hooded violet flowers look like an early military head-dress of the same name. It's a US native but is easy to grow in Britain. It has a long history of use as a sedative for anxiety, tension, hysteria, neuralgia, insomnia and other problems of the nervous system. As a natural tranquillizer, it can help reduce muscular tremors and tics, and some herbalists use it to treat drug withdrawal and delirium tremens (the shakes induced by overuse of alcohol). You can make it into an infusion or tincture for soothing nervous agitation (see Using Plants, page 34); take 3 times daily until symptoms pass.
NB If buying seeds or plugs, make sure you get the right species; Chinese skullcap (*S. baicalensis*) is a different plant.

GROWS/WHERE TO FIND
→ hardy perennial
→ likes sun
→ likes damp position
→ moisture-retentive soil
→ harvest leaves in early summer and dry for later use

Thyme
Thymus vulgaris

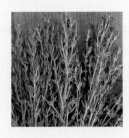

Thyme is a tiny plant, with leaves about 5 mm long and small, dense whorls of white-pink flowering spikes popping up in summer. It's traditionally used in *bouquets garnis* and many meat, fish and egg dishes. The essential oil contains thymol, which is an antiseptic and expectorant, and is often added to cough syrups and gargles to kill bacteria and loosen phlegm in the throat and chest. Try it as an antiseptic soap (see page 66) for use on sore or infected skin. Made into a salve or lotion, it can be topically applied to help soothe sore muscles and rheumatism. One laboratory study also showed that animals given thyme aged more slowly than others – but this anti-ageing effect has not yet been replicated in humans.
NB Use the oil sparingly in internal treatments because thymol is toxic in large doses.

To soothe aching muscles, fill a sterilized Kilner jar with the leaves and flowering tops of thyme, pour olive or almond oil over, and leave to steep for 2 weeks. Pour into a bath as needed.

GROWS/WHERE TO FIND
→ evergreen perennial
→ needs a sunny position – won't tolerate shade
→ gritty, free-draining soil
→ low-growing
→ harvest leaves and flowering tops for drying
→ replace after 3–4 years if plants become woody
→ buy fresh herb from supermarkets and essential oil from pharmacies

Wormwood
Artemisia absinthum

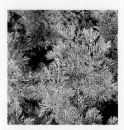

Wormwood is a native British and European plant with deeply cut silvery green leaves, bobbly yellow flowers and a very bitter flavour.
The 'bitters' in wormwood increase the production of bile and stomach acids and, taken as an infusion, can aid digestion, ease gas and bloating and increase appetite. Wormwood is also used as a tincture or tonic to improve the function of the liver and gall bladder.

The leaves and flowering shoots are strong insect-repellents (see Pest Pot-pourri, page 75) which can be dotted around the house, or made into a poultice (see Using Plants, page 36) to reduce swelling from insect stings and other skin inflammations.

NB Do not use if pregnant or breastfeeding. Do not take internally for longer than 2 weeks because a constituent of the oil, thujone, is toxic in large doses.

GROWS/WHERE TO FIND
→ perennial
→ likes poor, dry, well-drained soil
→ needs full sun
→ prop stems up with canes
→ collect leaves and flowerheads in summer for drying

FLOWERS AND LEAVES

Agrimony
Agrimonia eupatoria

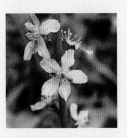

Agrimony's beautiful yellow flower spikes and toothed leaves can be seen along country lanes in summer. It's traditionally been used for liver complaints, including mild jaundice, and its bitter, anti-inflammatory properties can help with digestive problems such as diarrhoea and colitis. Nowadays, it's mostly known as a diuretic, which can soothe urinary tract disorders such as cystitis and irritable bladder. Take as a tea or tincture (see Using Plants, page 34), 3 times a day.

For recurrent cystitis, pack agrimony flowers and leaves into a Kilner jar and pour vodka over to cover, then seal and leave for 4–6 weeks in a dark place, shaking regularly. Strain and bottle. Take 4 drops in water, 3 times a day.

GROWS/WHERE TO FIND
→ perennial
→ hedgerows, roadsides, meadows
→ likes full sun
→ easy to grow
→ harvest flower spikes and leaves when in bloom for drying

Aloe
Aloe barbadensis

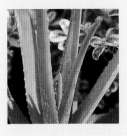

Although aloe is a tender succulent, you can grow it in pots indoors on a warm, sunny windowsill or conservatory during winter. It's a very handy first-aid remedy for burns, cuts and skin abrasions – just slice a leaf horizontally and apply the clear gel that oozes out of the centre directly on to the wound. Aloe gel has been shown to speed healing time and encourage cellular repair in burns, minor wounds, psoriasis and the scaly, red, flaking skin of seborrhoeic dermatitis. It can help skin recover from sunburn and frostbite and is often used in beauty treatments as a skin softener (see Beeswax Lip Balm, page 152). Its astringent properties may also help tighten skin and minimize wrinkles.

NB the clear gel from the inner leaves is different from the yellowish juice that comes from the tough outer edge of the leaves, and which is known as aloes when it has solidified. Aloes can cause intestinal cramping, so don't take orally.

GROWS/WHERE TO FIND
→ evergreen succulent
→ not hardy
→ grow in a pot in a sunny conservatory or on a window ledge
→ feed and put outdoors in summer
→ water sparingly in winter
→ cut leaves whenever needed and apply gel 2–4 times a day

Burdock
Arctium lappa* and *A. minus

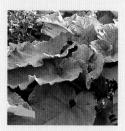

Burdock is sometimes called the 'Velcro plant', as the thistle-like burrs stick to anything that touches them.
It's a beautiful, tall biennial and its rosettes of large green leaves are used for infusions and poultices, while it has a long tap root that can be made into decoctions – mixed with dandelion root, it makes the classic dandelion and burdock. Burdock has long been used as a treatment for inflamed skin problems such as acne, boils, rashes, psoriasis, eczema and dermatitis. It's also helpful with the painful joints of gout and rheumatism.

To soothe skin eruptions, steam 2 burdock leaves, drain off excess water and quickly apply to the skin, as hot as you can stand. Cover with a bandage and place a warm (not hot) hot water bottle over the poultice, then leave on for 20 minutes.

GROWS/WHERE TO FIND
→ biennial
→ found in hedgerows, woodland edge and waste ground
→ flowers June–September
→ easy to grow
→ use roots in the second spring – they are long and can be hard to dig up

Chamomile
Matricaria recutita

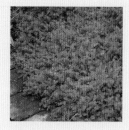

Known more as a pleasant-tasting tea than as a medicine, chamomile can be effective in health problems as diverse as indigestion, colic, inflamed skin, anxiety and poor sleep. It can be made into a cream for wounds, skin irritations, sore eyes (see Chamomile and Marigold Eye Lotion, page 147), nappy rash and to soothe sore nipples when breastfeeding.

It's also drunk as a tea to help with indigestion, colic, sciatica and gout. As a mild sedative and relaxant, it can help ease the anxiety and nervous stress that interferes with normal sleep function. Drink a cup 1 hour before bed, or add to a soothing bedtime bath (see Pom-pom Bath, page 80).

A first-rate remedy for children, chamomile tea can be safely given to infants and children from the age of 6 months upwards. For babies suffering from colic and digestive discomfort, breastfeeding mothers can drink the tea. It soothes fractious and over-tired infants, gently encouraging relaxation and a good night's sleep. It can also help with the pain of teething.

For a hair rinse, use chamomile tea as a final rinse to lighten blonde hair.

NB There are two kinds of chamomile, but the larger flowerheads of German chamomile (*Matricaria recutita*) are more popular in herbal remedies than Roman chamomile (*Chamaemelum nobile*).

GROWS/WHERE TO FIND
→ perennial
→ poor soil is best
→ prefers part-sun
→ self-seeds freely
→ collect flowerheads and dry

Chickweed
Stellaria media

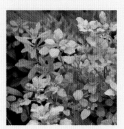

If you have a garden, you're bound to have encountered chickweed, one of the most ubiquitous weedy plants in Britain. It proliferates in quiet corners and empty spots, yet its delicate, white, star-shaped flowers are often a welcome sight as the first bloom of the year. Don't be tempted to dig up all your chickweed: this nutrient- and vitamin-rich plant has a wide range of beneficial properties, which are especially welcome during the colder months. Traditionally used in ointments to soothe itching and other inflamed skin conditions, chickweed is also a mild diuretic, and when drunk as a tea can help with rheumatism. The leaves have a mild, fruity taste and are delicious in salads – treat it as a cut-and-come-again wild green that'll keep your vitamin levels high during winter.

Chickweed Poultice: mash up leaves or make into an ointment (see Using Plants, page 35) and apply directly to soothe itching, eczema, psoriasis, boils or sunburn.

GROWS/WHERE TO FIND
→ winter annual
→ weed found in moist soil, beds and lawns
→ blooms late winter to spring
→ use young leaves in salads

Cinquefoil
Potentilla reptans

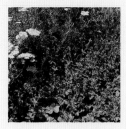

The lobes on the leaves of this common garden weed look like the fingers of an outspread hand – 'cinquefoil' is derived from the Latin, *quinquefolium*, meaning five leaves. It's an invasive plant with running stems over 1 m long, and small buttercup-like yellow flowers. Infusions of the leaves and roots have a long history of use in traditional medicine to treat fever, diarrhoea, toothache and mouth ulcers. Cinquefoil has astringent properties; when made into a lotion for the skin, it is often said to help 'tighten' tissues for an anti-ageing effect. Pick cinquefoil from the wild rather than introducing into your garden – it can spread voraciously.

For toothache and mouth ulcers, infuse 30 g fresh leaves in 500 ml freshly boiled water, then cover and leave for 10 minutes. Strain and cool. Use to gargle, swishing round the mouth for 60 seconds, then spit. Use the gargle 3–4 times a day.

GROWS/WHERE TO FIND
→ perennial
→ likes sun
→ invasive, colonizing by runners
→ best to pick from the wild
→ flowers June–September

Daisy
Bellis perennis

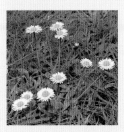

The common daisy is one of the most pervasive lawn invaders, so it's satisfying to know that its ever-flowering white-pink blooms can be put to some good use. Daisy has traditionally been thought of as a good wound healer and, when made into a salve (see Using Plants, page 35), can soothe cuts, sores, bruises and stiff joints. Made into an infusion or gargle, the flowers and leaves have long been used to help with all manner of respiratory tract infections, including coughs, catarrh, bronchitis and sinusitis. Daisy tea is also reputed to be a pick-me-up for listlessness and low energy.

GROWS/WHERE TO FIND
→ evergreen perennial
→ found in lawns
→ likes sun
→ flowers throughout the year
→ use flowerheads and leaves fresh or dried

Elderflower
Sambucus nigra

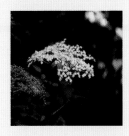

Creamy clusters of elderflowers arrive in June and July, and are often used to make cordials and elderflower wine – traditionally drunk hot as a remedy for colds and flu. Elderflowers, like elderberries (see page 161), have antiviral properties that can help combat flu, making symptoms less severe and speeding up the rate of recovery. Take regular infusions as soon as you feel the first signs of infection.

Elderflower is also a good inflammatory and decongestant. Made into a cough remedy, it can soothe sore throats, coughs and bronchial infections, and make catarrh and sinus conditions looser and more productive.

GROWS/WHERE TO FIND
→ deciduous shrub or tree, considered a 'weed'
→ found in wasteland, hedgerows, beside paths
→ likes sun but shade-tolerant
→ flowers June–July
→ use only fresh, cream-coloured flowers, before they turn brown

Feverfew
Tanacetum parthenium

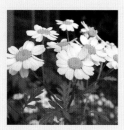

Feverfew has been used to lower fevers and as a headache cure since the 17th century. But it wasn't until 1974, when a Welsh doctor's wife apparently cured herself of chronic migraines by eating a few feverfew leaves each day, that it became known as a treatment for migraine. A flurry of clinical studies followed, and feverfew is now widely used to prevent and lessen the severity of chronic migraines. It can reduce the duration of migraine headaches, decreasing pain, vomiting and sensitivity to light. Taken regularly, feverfew also seems to make migraine attacks less frequent.

However, the leaves taste very bitter and some people find them slightly nauseating. You can disguise the taste in sandwiches (see Feverfew Sandwiches, page 122; the butter helps counteract the bitterness) or in a big plate of mixed salad leaves.

For a Feverfew Tea, brew 30 g fresh feverfew leaves in 50 ml freshly boiled water, then cover and leave for 10 minutes. Strain. Drink 1 cup daily, adding honey, sugar or lemon to taste. NB Fresh feverfew leaves can cause swelling and soreness in the mouth. Discontinue if this happens and do not use during pregnancy.

GROWS/WHERE TO FIND
→ perennial
→ likes sun
→ drought-tolerant
→ self-seeds prolifically
→ flowers June–August
→ use fresh leaves
→ for drying, harvest whole plant when flowering

Fleabane
Erigeron karvinskianus

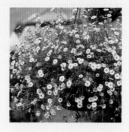

Native Americans burned fleabane to ward off fleas and other pests, which is probably where its common name originated. Today, this pretty daisy-like flower is a prolific weed, but one with significant herbal uses. It's diuretic and astringent, helping tissues tighten and contract, and has traditionally been used in the treatment of kidney disorders, diarrhoea and menstrual problems. One study showed fleabane lowered blood pressure temporarily in animals, and it has been used to help stop the flow of blood in minor haemorrhages such as nosebleeds. The leaves and flowers can be infused and drunk as a tea (see Using Plants, page 34).

Fleabane Pet Bedding: dry leaves and flowers, then crumble and put in a small muslin bag. Place among your pet's bedding. Worth a try!

GROWS/WHERE TO FIND
→ annual and perennial weed
→ likes light soils and sunny spots, eg rock gardens
→ bountiful daisy-like flower-heads from spring to autumn
→ use leaves and flowers

Honeysuckle Flower
Lonicera periclymenum

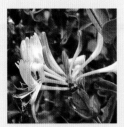

One of the most fragrant garden plants, honeysuckle is also used as a remedy for respiratory illnesses. The flowers are rich in salicylic acid, which has painkilling properties, and can be helpful with sore throats, headaches, bronchial complaints, croup, rheumatism and arthritis. Drink as a tea or gargle with for best effects. It's also a cooling plant and can calm fever, hot flushes and sunstroke.

Honeysuckle Honey: place washed flowers and buds in a jar, leaving a 2 cm gap at the top. Cover completely with runny honey, then seal and leave to steep for 2 weeks (check that the flowers are always covered, or they may go mouldy). Strain and bottle in a sterilized container. Take 2 tsp a day.

GROWS/WHERE TO FIND
→ deciduous shrub
→ likes dappled shade
→ prone to mildew (don't allow to dry out, as mildew will set in)
→ climber that needs support
→ flowers June–August
→ use flowers fresh or dried

Lady's Mantle
Alchemilla xanthochlora

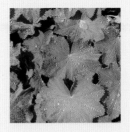

The contrast of the acid-yellow flowers and dark green leaves of lady's mantle make it a stunning ground cover plant in cottage-type gardens. When it blooms from June to September, cut the flowering stems and leaves and dry for use in herbal remedies. Lady's mantle contains essential compounds that, applied externally to wounds, stop bleeding by clotting the blood. You can make it into a salve for use with cuts and wounds and it's also helpful for stopping general itchiness of the skin.

Made into a tea, lady's mantle is often used to combat excessive menstrual bleeding and diarrhoea. Its coagulant properties appear to decrease menstrual blood flow and vaginal discharge after a few weeks' use. The tea can also be used as a mouthwash for bleeding gums, especially after dental procedures.

To help with heavy menstrual bleeding, make an infusion with 30 g dried leaves and flowering stems in 500 ml freshly boiled water. Cover and leave to steep for 10 minutes. Drink a cup 3 times a day.

GROWS/WHERE TO FIND
→ perennial
→ slow growing
→ good ground cover
→ likes dappled sun
→ flowers June–September
→ harvest leaves and flowering stems for drying

Lavender
Lavandula angustifolia

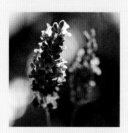

Lavender has been used in bathing since Roman times; in fact, the Latin *lavare,* from which lavender takes its name, means 'to wash'. With its powerful but calming scent, lavender is now used in a huge range of perfumes, cosmetics and soaps. The essential oil in the flowers has a soothing, sedative effect, which calms nerves, relaxes muscles, eases anxiety and helps promote sleep. You can use it as an inhalation or in baths (see Lavender Bath Bomb, page 139), or make it into a gently antiseptic salve for cuts and bruises, to help minimize scarring and relieve skin irritations.

Taken as a tea or tincture (see Using Plants, page 34), lavender has soothing effects on the central nervous system generally. It's thought to slow nerve reactions, slightly easing pain and irritability and clearing the mind of nervous tension. It can help with sleeping difficulties; a cup of lavender tea about 1 hour before bed acts as a mild sedative for insomnia. Lavender also aids digestion, relieving intestinal spasms and quelling 'nervous' stomach complaints.

GROWS/WHERE TO FIND
→ evergreen shrub
→ needs full sun
→ likes poor, gritty soil
→ good for pots
→ for drying, harvest flowers from mid- to late summer, when petals are just opening
→ clip back after flowering; don't cut into old wood
→ buy lavender essential oil from health food shops

Marigold
Calendula officinalis

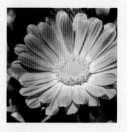

The bright orange marigold may no longer be a very fashionable flower but it's still extremely useful medicinally, having antiseptic and anti-inflammatory properties and a wealth of potential uses. As a lotion, cream, or ointment, it will speed up healing and counter infection in conditions as diverse as minor burns and sunburn, insect bites and stings, sore and pustular spots, acne (see Marigold, Lavender and Rose Geranium Gel, page 64), cuts and abrasions, inflamed rashes such as nappy rash, and haemorrhoids and varicose veins.

Taken as a tea or tincture (see Using Plants, page 34), it helps soothe stomach disorders and ulcers and is also used in the treatment of extremely painful periods, known as dysmenorrhoea. Only the flowerheads are used: harvest them as they bloom.
NB When using Marigolds it is important to choose plants from the genus known as *Calendula*. Trickily in horticulture, most 'marigolds' are actually from an entirely different species known as *Tagetes*. If in doubt do check with your stockist, as the medicinal properties of the two species are very different.

GROWS/WHERE TO FIND
→ annual
→ easy to grow from seed and available as plants early in summer bedding season
→ prefers full sun
→ good in containers and window boxes
→ harvest flowers; deadhead regularly to keep plants flowering

Motherwort
Leonurus cardiaca

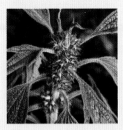

The tall, raggedy, sometimes fluffy flowering stems of motherwort grows wild on wasteland across the country. It's easy to grow in the garden too and, at 1.5 m tall, makes an interesting addition at the back of a herbaceous border. The flowering stems are traditionally used as a heart tonic, the plant's slightly sedative effect soothing palpitations and nervous irritability. It doesn't make you drowsy, just calmer and more relaxed.

Motherwort, as you can guess from the name, has also been used with premenstrual syndrome, to minimize pain, bloating, anxiety and irritability. It contracts the womb and improves blood flow, so can be used to hurry along late periods. However, it shouldn't be used by women who already have heavy bleeds or those who may have an underlying undiagnosed disorder. Motherwort can be taken as a tea but it doesn't taste pleasant. Try it as a tincture or make into a honey instead (see Using Plants, pages 34 and 36). NB Do not use during pregnancy.

GROWS/WHERE TO FIND
→ found in wasteground
→ grows easily from seed
→ likes poor soil
→ harvest flowering stems in August when in full bloom

Mullein
Verbascum thapsus

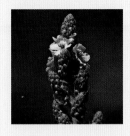

This statuesque plant has long been a staple in herbal medicine, used as an expectorant, decongestant and mucus reducer for catarrh and to ease chest complaints such as bronchitis. The leaves, made into a lotion or ointment, aid wound healing and soothe inflammation, and the infused oil makes an excellent treatment for earache caused by compacted wax (see Wax-dissolving Drops, page 82). Mullein grows wild, but its dramatic yellow, spiked flowers and felted, greeny-silver rosettes of foliage look fantastic in any garden. Collect wild seeds or buy and scatter during spring/autumn.

Mullein Tea: pick 5–6 large green leaves during the flowering season (the small hairs on the leaves can irritate the skin, so wear gardening gloves). Wash, then chop and place in a teapot. Add 500 ml hot water and leave to steep for 10 mins. Strain. Drink for irritations of throat and chest.

GROWS/WHERE TO FIND
→ grows wild and in gardens
→ biennial, dying back after 2 years
→ best in well-drained soil
→ likes full sun
→ self-seeds easily
→ flowers early summer
→ may need staking

Nasturtium
Tropaeolum majus

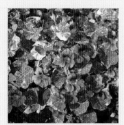

These colourful flowers have a surprisingly zingy flavour and are used to brighten up the look *and* taste of summer salads. Nasturtium has other benefits too: the flowers and leaves have antimicrobial properties and are used to treat bronchitis, catarrh and bacterial infections of the upper respiratory tract. The plant's active compounds seem to help loosen and clear phlegm, making breathing easier. Nasturtium can made into a tincture, honey or vinegar (see Using Plants, pages 34 and 36). As a tea, it can be drunk, used as a gargle for infected throats, or as a gently antiseptic face wash for spot-prone skin.

To ease catarrh, try nasturtium vinegar. Place 1 cup flowers/leaves in a bottle with 1 garlic clove, then pour over 500 ml cider vinegar to cover completely (otherwise the flowers may go mouldy). Seal and leave for 4 weeks. Strain, bottle and take 1 tsp twice a day.

GROWS/WHERE TO FIND
→ annual
→ can be grown in containers
→ likes sun
→ self-seeds readily
→ harvest leaves and flowers in summer and use fresh

Nettle
Urtica dioica

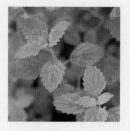

The stinging nettle might not be our most loved plant, but it's certainly one of the most useful. Nettle leaves are very nutritious, high in vitamins, minerals and chlorophyll. When made into soups or eaten raw (be brave, but roll them up in a tight ball first), they can give the immune system a boost at any time of year (see Nettle Soup and Pesto, page 114). They contain anti-inflammatories and natural painkillers and have a long history of treating rheumatic disorders and arthritis. Recent research illustrates the point: applied as a lotion to sore joints or drunk as a tea, nettles appear to reduce the pain of arthritis and lessen the need for painkillers like aspirin and ibuprofen.

The yellow roots provide treatment for an enlarged prostate, a condition that affects many men in midlife. After taking nettle root extract for a few months, both urine flow and frequency were shown to improve.

You can also add a nettle rinse to your haircare routine to help dandruff, improve growth, and bring a healthy, glossy shine to hair (see page 128).

To ease the pain of acute arthritis, steep 50 g fresh young nettle tops in 500 ml freshly boiled water. Cover and leave for 10 minutes. Strain, Makes 3 cups to be drunk over the day.

GROWS/WHERE TO FIND
→ in wasteland, banks, hedgerows, woods
→ prefers nitrogen-rich soil
→ harvest the top 15 cm of young tops in spring (wear gloves)
→ tops will quickly regrow and can be cut again throughout season
→ harvest roots in autumn
→ buy root extract from pharmacies

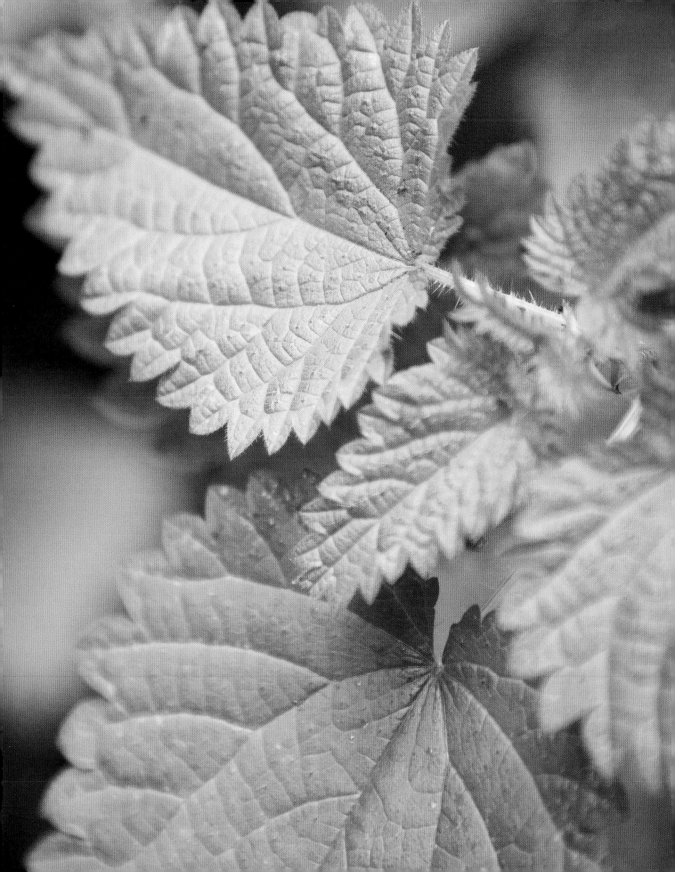

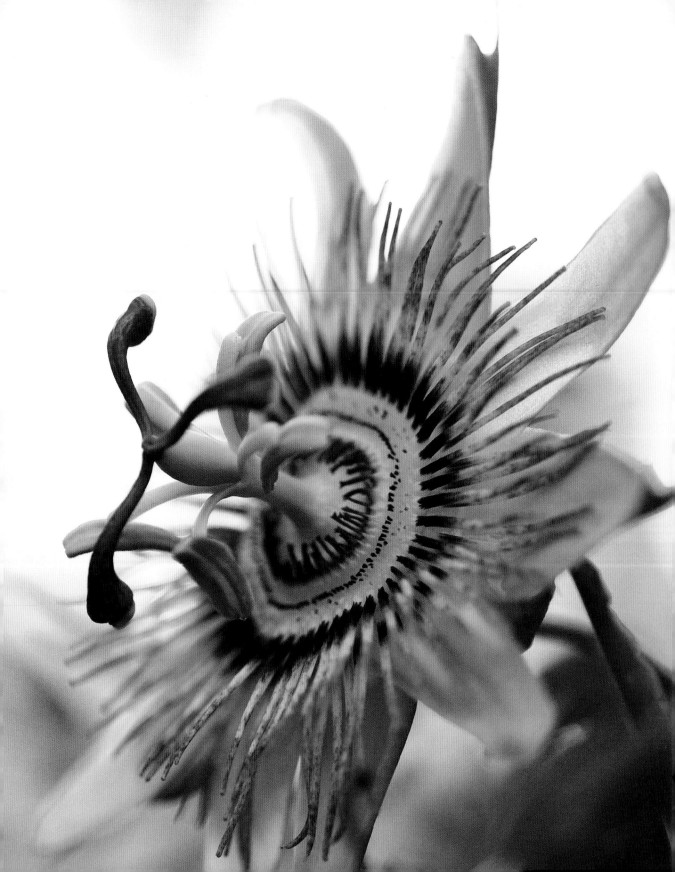

Passion Flower
Passiflora **spp.**

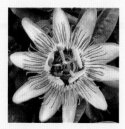

The dramatic showy blooms of passion flower and its leaves have a calming, sedative effect when made into teas and tinctures. Passion flower is often used to treat anxiety, to soothe tension and restlessness, lower blood pressure and help with sleeping problems arising from nervous distress. It can also help settle nervous stomach disorders.

For Passion Flower Tea, infuse a few leaves or flower petals in freshly boiled water and drink as a tea, 3 times a day.

GROWS/WHERE TO FIND
→ climber
→ likes poor, sandy soil
→ will grow outdoors in the south in a sunny, protected site
→ in colder locations, grow in a greenhouse or conservatory
→ restrict roots to encourage fruiting
→ provide support
→ use flowers fresh or dried

Red Clover
Trifolium pratense

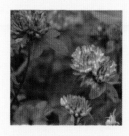

Red clover is found in the wild and used by farmers as a soil improver and forage crop. In recent years, the flowers have received a lot of attention as a natural form of hormone replacement therapy for the menopause. Red clover is high in isoflavones, phytoestrogenic compounds that are thought to help reduce hot flushes, night sweats and other symptoms of menopause, as well as premenstrual syndrome (PMS). But, as yet, no large clinical studies have confirmed its usefulness in either the menopause or PMS.

Red clover is best taken as a tea made from the dried flowers (see Using Plants, page 34).

GROWS/WHERE TO FIND
→ perennial
→ found in meadows, paths, woods
→ likes loamy soil
→ easy to grow
→ harvest open flowerheads for drying

Rose Geranium
Pelargonium graveolens

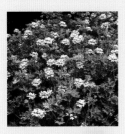

This tender, rose-scented geranium isn't frost-hardy and won't last long outside, but can be potted and kept indoors in a cool, light room or conservatory. It's worth it for the wonderful aroma – the essential oil has slightly minty undertones and is very popular in aromatherapy – and both flowers and leaves can be dried and used in pot-pourri.

In remedies, rose geranium is often used as a balm to soothe acne (see Marigold, Lavender and Rose Geranium Gel, page 64), eczema and other skin conditions. It has antiseptic and anti-inflammatory properties, and was traditionally used as a tea or tincture to treat nausea, tonsillitis and poor circulation. Pour the infusion (see Using Plants, page 34) into the bath to soothe skin – you'll definitely come out smelling of roses.

GROWS/WHERE TO FIND

→ evergreen shrub
→ not fully hardy
→ pot and keep indoors
→ water sparingly
→ cut back annually to stop plants getting leggy
→ harvest fresh leaves all year
→ buy essential oil from pharmacies

Self-heal
Prunella vulgaris

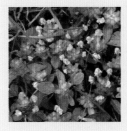

You find this pretty, low-growing plant in meadows and woods, its intensely violet flowers on spikes, with two bracts looking almost like a collar underneath. It's renowned as a wound healer, calming inflammation and helping to stop blood flow, hence its other names: heal-all, woundwort and hock heal. Make it into a salve for first-aid use on cuts, burns, bruises, ulcers, bites, cold sores (see below) and minor injuries.

Self-heal also has antiviral properties and, taken internally as a tea or tincture (see Using Plants, page 34), can help with throat infections, flu and fever. It's been shown to hinder the ability of some viruses (including the cold sore virus) to replicate. The tea can also be used as a gargle for inflamed gums, mouth ulcers and to soothe sore throats.

For a skin soother, pack a sterilized Kilner jar with fresh self-heal flowers and leaves, and pour over enough olive oil to cover. Seal, and leave on a sunny window ledge for 3–4 weeks, or until all colour has leached from the plants. Strain, then bottle. Apply to affected area twice daily, or use as a bath oil.

GROWS/WHERE TO FIND

→ ground-cover perennial
→ invasive by creeping underground stems
→ grow in wildflower meadow
→ cut flowering stems in summer for drying

St John's Wort
Hypericum perforatum

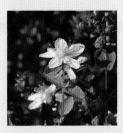

The yellow flowers of St John's wort provide a natural antidepressant. The herb has been used for centuries to treat the age-old disorders of melancholy and hysteria. But in the last 30 years it's been proved as effective in the treatment of mild to moderate depression as prescribed antidepressants – and without many of the side effects. The plant contains hypericin and hyperforin, active compounds that help relieve anxiety, depression, nervous tension, seasonal affective disorder (SAD) and insomnia. Make the flowers into a tea or tincture (see Using Plants, page 34) and take daily.

St John's wort also has a very long history of use as a wound healer. When made into a salve, its anti-inflammatory properties help soothe cuts, bruises and inflamed skin (see Jelly Balm, page 73). It's also known as an antiviral, which can help with herpes and hepatitis.
NB Do not take St John's wort if you are on any medication without checking with your doctor or pharmacist – particularly the Pill, antidepressants or warfarin.

GROWS/WHERE TO FIND
→ perennial
→ likes sun
→ good meadow plant
→ self-seeds profusely
→ summer-flowering
→ harvest flowering tops and use fresh or dry

Vervain
Verbena officinalis

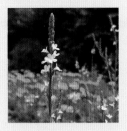

It's unusual to see the delicate, lilac flowering spikes of vervain in the wild nowadays, but it's so pretty and reputed to be such a cure-all that it's definitely worth growing in the garden. Like self-heal, it has an astonishing range of applications, and is used for insomnia, depression, headaches, hot flushes, coughs, chronic fatigue and problems with digestion. It's perhaps most useful as a nerve soother, restoring calm after periods of nervous tension or physical exhaustion, and thus helping to improve sleep and lift mood. It can make you sweat, so is used to bring down temperature, and has anti-inflammatory and painkilling properties, so it can help with headaches and premenstrual syndrome. Its bitter and laxative properties make it useful for digestive problems. Take as an infusion made from fresh or dried flowering stems and leaves (see Using Plants, page 34). It can also be applied to the skin to treat burns, inflammation and wounds.

GROWS/WHERE TO FIND
→ perennial
→ likes lime soil
→ harvest late in the flowering season for drying

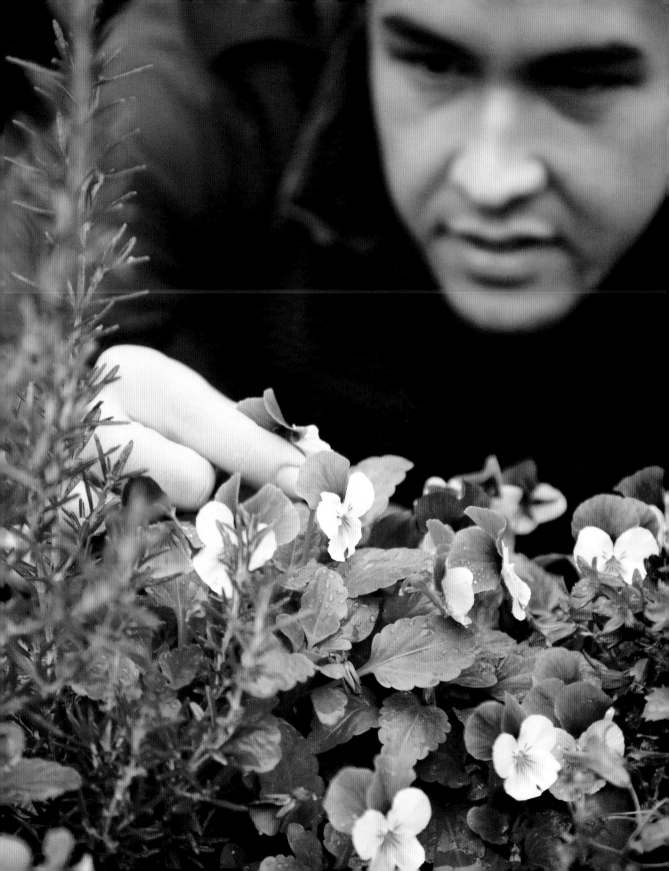

Viola
Viola tricolor

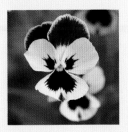

Known as hearts-ease or wild pansy, this tiny plant grows wild and is also cultivated in gardens for its long flowering season. It is an anti-inflammatory and has traditionally been used as a soothing balm for eczema (see Viola and Chamomile Cream, page 56), acne, pustular spots and other skin outbreaks. Taken as a tea (see Using Plants, page 34), it can loosen congestion in bronchitis and coughs, and its diuretic properties also help with cystitis, rheumatism and urinary disorders.

GROWS/WHERE TO FIND
→ small perennial often treated as an annual
→ easy to grow from seed
→ likes semi-shade
→ flowers April–September
→ harvest throughout flowering season and use fresh or dried

Woodruff
Galium odoratum

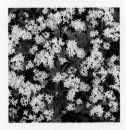

This woodland plant, often found nestling in moist patches beneath trees, smells of freshly mown hay – an aroma that only intensifies when the flowering parts are dried. It makes a delicious tea (see Using Plants, page 34), which is traditionally used as a tonic to boost liver function and help with arthritis. It's a mild sedative and can soothe agitation, restlessness and anxiety, helping to improve disordered sleep and insomnia.

GROWS/WHERE TO FIND
→ perennial
→ good ground cover
→ likes moist soil
→ likes shade
→ invasive
→ flowers late spring/early summer
→ harvest just before flowering and use dried for best flavour

Yarrow
Achillea millefolium

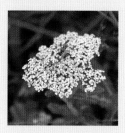

Yarrow is also known as woundwort, nosebleed, staunchweed and bloodwort and was traditionally packed into open wounds to staunch bleeding. As a salve or lotion (see Using Plants, page 35), it can be used to stop bleeding cuts and wounds, and to improve the healing of bruises, rashes and piles.

Versatile yarrow has many other medicinal properties too. Drunk as a hot tea, it brings down temperature and encourages sweating, so is helpful for colds, flu, catarrh, rheumatism and fever. The essential oil can be made into a chest rub for bronchial complaints and coughs. The tea has a bitter astringency (add sugar to taste), which helps soothe digestion and stop diarrhoea. Yarrow can also lower blood pressure slightly and, as it contains the painkiller salicylic acid, is useful for headaches, menstrual cramps and the pain of arthritis.
NB Don't use during pregnancy.

To staunch nosebleeds, bruise and roll a few fresh yarrow leaves into a ball and plug into the affected nostril. Gently remove once bleeding has stopped.

GROWS/WHERE TO FIND
→ perennial
→ grows wild in meadows and hedgerows
→ easy to grow
→ likes sun
→ flowers June–September
→ harvest flowers and leaves while in bloom for drying
→ buy essential oil from pharmacies

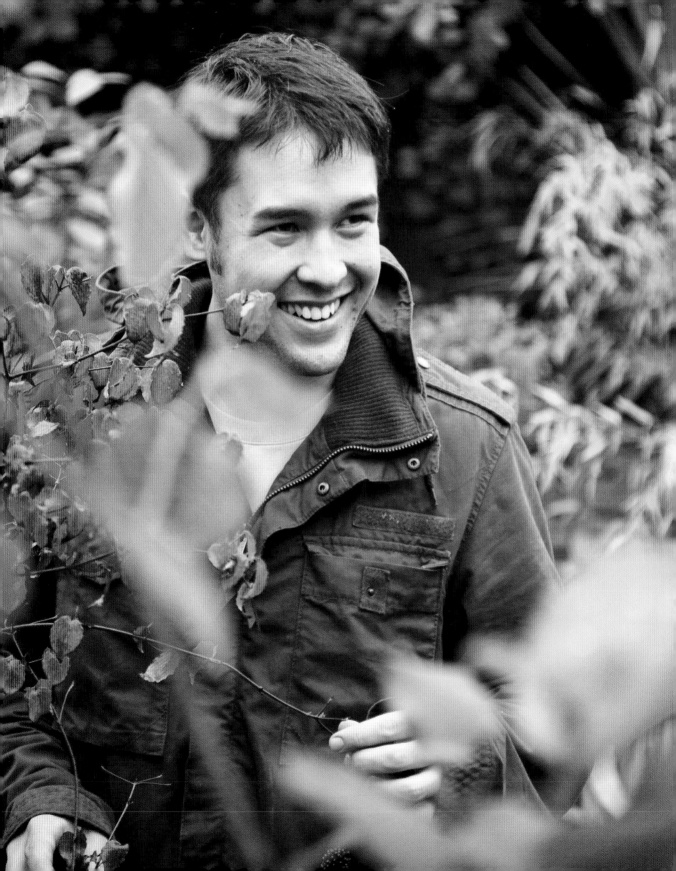

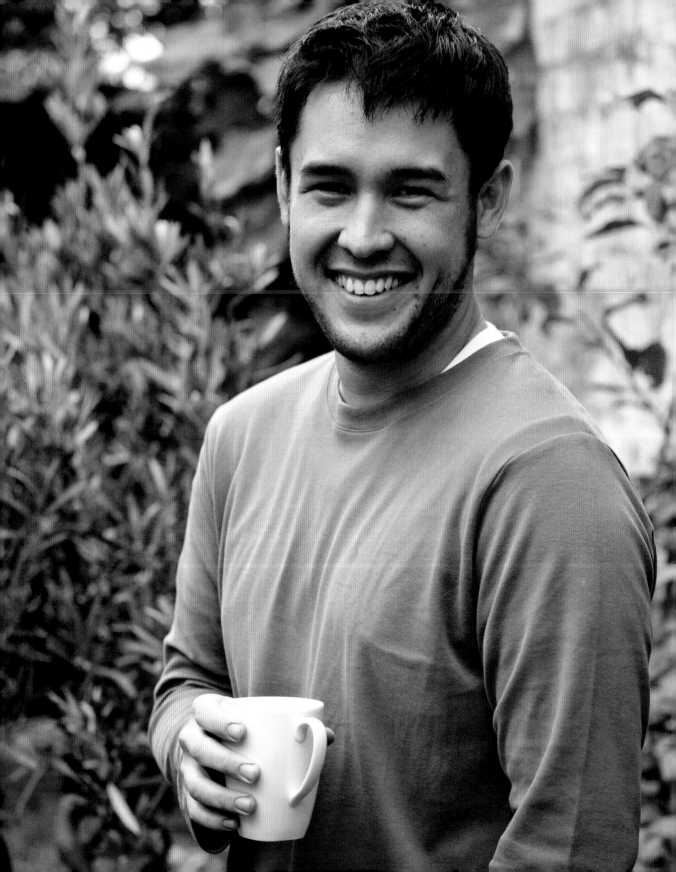

RESOURCES

STOCKISTS

Most of the equipment and plant material you'll need is easily available in kitchen, hardware and gardening stores. Here are a few suppliers who stock more specialist items.

G. BALDWIN & CO.
020 7703 5550 www.baldwins.co.uk
Shop and online shop
Bottles and jars, pump/drop dispensers, beeswax, emulsifying wax, resin, Irish moss, essential oils.

BARWINNOCK HERBS
01465 821338 www.barwinnock.com
Nursery and online shop. Based in Ayrshire, Scotland.

HARPTREE NURSERY
01761 221370 www.harptreenursery.co.uk
Nursery and online shop. Based in Bath.

HERBS FOR HEALING
01285 851457 www.herbsforhealing.net
Online shop. Beeswax, jars, muslin, funnels, herbs. Based in Gloucester.

JEKKA'S HERB FARM
01454 418878 www.jekkasherbfarm.com
Online shop. Large selection of plants and seeds.

LAUREL FARM HERBS
01728 668223 www.laurelfarmherbs.co.uk
Nursery and online shop. Based in Suffolk.

LIMEBURN NURSERIES
01275 333399 www.arneherbs.co.uk
Nursery and online shop. Based in Bristol.

NEAL'S YARD REMEDIES
0845 262 3145 www.nealsyardremedies.co.uk
Shops and online. Bottles and jars, pump/drop dispensers, beeswax, emulsifying wax, essential oils.

NORFOLK HERBS
01362 860812 www.norfolkherbs.co.uk
Nursery and online shop. Based in Norfolk.

SPICE WORLD
01984 633685 www.spiceworld.uk.com
Online shop. Wide range of medicinal herbs and organic products.

PLANT INFORMATION

BOTANIC GARDENS CONSERVATION INTERNATIONAL
www.bgci.org
A global network of botanic gardens working for plant conservation and undertaking medicinal plant research around the world.

BOTANICAL SOCIETY OF THE BRITISH ISLES
www.bsbi.org.uk
Society offers flora maps, plant identification guides, archives of botanical publications.

THE HERB SOCIETY
www.herbsociety.org.uk
Detailed information on the medicinal, culinary and historical uses of herbs.

NATURAL ENGLAND
www.naturalengland.org.uk
News on English wildlife and conservation efforts.

PLANTLIFE INTERNATIONAL
www.plantlife.org.uk
Organization staging countrywide events to promote the defence of wildlife and natural reserves.

RHS PLANT FINDER
www.rhs.org.uk
Database of plant information and gardening advice, with a nursery-finder tool.

THE WILDLIFE TRUSTS
www.wildlifetrusts.org
Foundation dedicated to conserving the full range of the UK's natural habitat and wildlife.

INDEX

ACKNOWLEDGEMENTS

AUTHOR'S ACKNOWLEDGEMENTS

Working on this TV series and book has been a huge adventure. Behind the scenes there has been a whole team of people whose untiring efforts have helped make it all possible. Firstly, a huge thank you is in order to Lisa Edwards at the BBC for taking a chance on the idea. Equally, all the team at Silver River (you know who you are) have been absolutely brilliant. I've never seen such passion and dedication, particularly when following me around wet fields in the cold rain! Liz at the University of Reading has been a true star with her pharmaceutical genius, and of course a huge thank you to my agent Fiona for her unending patience. I am also greatly indebted to HarperCollins for putting together this brilliant book. I had great fun working on it with them. Lastly, a major thanks to all my family and friends for believing in me – and putting up with my geeky plant obsession for all these years.

PUBLISHERS' ACKNOWLEDGEMENTS

The publishers would like to thank Timothy Dunn of Timothy Dunn Florists for a fabulous selection of flowers; Ginkgo Gardens for their help with photography; Peter Jarrett, of Middlesex University, for providing photographs from the university's Herbal Medicine Garden; and Kathryn Lwin Brooks of the Archway Clinic of Herbal Medicine.

PICTURE CREDITS

All photographs other than those listed below have been provided by Noel Murphy. Bailey-Cooper Photography 3/Alamy Stock Photo 105; Garden Picture Library 180R, 181L, 191L, 212L; iStock 157L, 159R, 174L, 185R, 187, 207L; Peter Jarrett (Medicinal Herb Garden of Middlesex University) 159L, 161R, 177R, 179R, 184L, 185L, 194R, 197L, 200L, 204L, 213R; Shutterstock 157R, 160L, 161L, 165R, 166L, 166R, 167L, 168R, 169R, 170, 171L, 173, 189L, 190L, 190R, 191R, 193R, 194L, 196R, 203R, 205R, 206R, 207R, 211L, 215L, 215R; William Shaw 162R, 168L.